Humanhood

Also by Joseph Fletcher

The Church and Industry (1930)
Christianity and Property (1947)
Morals and Medicine (1954)
Situation Ethics (1966)
Moral Responsibility (1967)
The Situation Ethics Debate (1968)
    (with Harvey Cox)
Hello Lovers (1970)
    (with Thomas Wassmer, SJ)
The Ethics of Genetic Control (1974)

Humanhood:
Essays in
Biomedical Ethics

JOSEPH FLETCHER

fB *Prometheus Books*
1203 Kensington Avenue
Buffalo, New York 14215

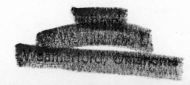

Essay Index

Published 1979 by Prometheus Books
1203 Kensington Avenue, Buffalo, New York 14215

Library of Congress Catalog Number: 79-1756
ISBN 0-87975-112-6

Printed in the United States of America

To our grandchildren:
Julia, Tom, and Edward.

Acknowledgments

Grateful acknowledgement is made to the following for permission to make use of earlier essays, in part or in full:

"Humanhood," from "Medicine and the Nature of Man," in *The Teaching of Medical Ethics*, ed. Robert M. Veatch, Willard Gaylin, and Councilman Morgan (Hastings-on-Hudson, New York: Institute of Society, Ethics and the Life Sciences, 1973), 47-58.

"Happiness," from "Being Happy, Being Human," *The Humanist*, 35:1, (January-February 1975) 13-15.

"Goodness," from "Virtue is a Pedicate," *The Monist* 54:1 (January 1970) 66-85.

"Distributive Justice," from "Ethics and Health Care Delivery," in *Ethics and Health Policy*, ed. Robert M. Veatch and Roy Branson, (Cambridge, Massachusetts: Ballinger Publishing Company [Lippincott], 1976) 99-109.

"Sharing With Others," from "Give If It Helps But Not If It Hurts," in *World Hunger and Moral Obligation*, ed. William Aiken and Hugh LaFollette (Englewood Cliffs, New Jersey: Prentice-Hall, Inc., 1977) 103-114.

"Wasting Human Bodies," from "Our Shameful Waste of Human Tissue," in *Updating Life and Death*, ed. Donald R. Cutler (Boston: Beacon Press, 1968) 1-30.

"Genetic Engineering," from "Ethical Aspects of Genetic Controls," *The New England Journal of Medicine* 285 (September 30, 1971) 776-783.

"Fetal Research," from "Fetal Research: An Ethical Appraisal," in *Appendix: Research on the Fetus* (Washington, D.C.: National Commission for the Protection of Health, Education, and Welfare Publication No. (OS) 76-188, 1975), 3-1 to 3-14.

"Abortion," from *The Ethics of Genetic Control,* Joseph Fletcher (New York: Doubleday and Company, 1974), 132-146.

"Infanticide," from "Infanticide and the Ethics of Loving Concern," in *Infanticide and the Value of Life,* ed. Marvin Kohl (Buffalo, New York: Prometheus Books, 1978), 13-22.

"Euthanasia," from "Ethics and Euthanasia," in *To Live and To Die*, ed. Robert H. Williams (New York: Springer-Verlag, 1973), 113-122.

"Cerebration," from "New Definitions of Death," in *Prism (AMA),* 2 (January 1974) 1, 13-14, 36.

"Suicide," from "In Verteigigung des Suizids," in *Suizid und Euthanasie,* ed. Albin Eser (Stuttgart: Ferdinand Enke Verlag, 1976), 233-244.

"Experiments on Humans," from "Ethical Considerations in Biomedical Research Involving Human Beings," in *Proceedings of the International Conference on the Role of the Individual and the Community in the Research, Development and Use of Biologicals (Geneva, 2-5 March, 1976)* (Geneva: World Health Organization, 1977) 101-110.

"Recombining DNA," from "Ethics and Recombinant DNA Research," in *The Southern California Law Review,* 1978 (51:6).

Contents

Introduction   xii

Author's Preface   1

Chapter 1. Humanness   7

         2. Happiness   20

         3. Goodness   27

         4. Distributive Justice   41

         5. Sharing with Others   54

         6. Wasting Human Bodies   65

         7. Genetic Engineering   79

         8. Fetal Research   93

         9. Our Duty to the Unborn   106

       10. Abortion   132

       11. Infanticide   140

       12. Euthanasia   149

       13. Cerebration   159

       14. Suicide   166

       15. Experiments on Humans   176

       16. Recombining DNA   190

Index   200

Introduction

I first met Joseph Fletcher about ten years ago, when he came to the University of Virginia to read a paper in the auditorium of the School of Medicine, and I was captivated by his enthusiasm and warmth immediately. Subsequently, during his years in residence at the University of Virginia as Visiting Professor of Medical Ethics, and more recently on a part-time basis, we have spent countless hours together with faculty and students from all parts of the University, educating each other across the boundaries of our collective uncertainties. My exposure to the literature and thought of writers in the field of ethics had been pitifully small.

Dr. Fletcher had written *Morals and Medicine* in 1954 from the Robert Treat Paine chair in Social Ethics at the Episcopal Theological School in Cambridge, Massachusetts, but he knew much more about morals, of course, than he did about medicine. He was aware of this, and set about finding out as much as he could about biologists, doctors, nurses, medical students, and all of the complex mix of people and science that go to make modern biology and medicine tick.

Not a scientist, he has brainstormed with many of the best of them. As a result of exchanges with Garrett Hardin, Joshua Lederberg, Robert Sinsheimer, Bernard Davis, Robert Wagner, and many, many others, his horizons in biology have expanded considerably. And, unlike many ethicists, he has spent much time with doctors and patients in a wide variety of institutions from one end of the country to the other.

His basic stance philosophically is that of a humanist, and his ethics are consequentialist. That is, he believes that human acts are fundamentally justified by the balance of their consequences, long run as well as short run, as measured in human values. In cutting loose from moral rules, as he has done in *Situation Ethics*, he emphasizes the essential human quality of reasoned choice as basic to morality. To follow a rule no matter what the result is in his book immoral and is an abdication of one's human responsibility. This position frightens many people who see it as an abandonment of principles and a dangerous venture on to the "slippery slope." Long term consequences are often imponderable and man cannot be trusted to appraise each situation adequately. True, he says, but what is needed are guidelines, not rules, and if we are to become truly human we must accept the uncertainty and assume the responsibility for our moral choices. It is not enough to look up the rule in the book and follow it.

Where does this lead us? The reader of these essays, which cover many of the most controversial issues in biomedical ethics, will have to judge for himself. Dr. Fletcher does not have the final answer to any of these questions he analyses. He knows, as many seem not to, that answers to value questions are susceptible neither of proof nor of disproof in a scientific sense. But like most scientists, he has faith in man's ability to better his condition through reason and by following the path of *agape* or loving concern. He further believes that knowledge is preferable to ignorance, dangerous though it may sometimes seem; this makes him a friend of research.

Finally, he is not afraid of controversy. He is willing to take a position for the sake of opening up discussion, as exemplified by his essay on "Humanhood" which first tackled one of the central issues in medical ethics: What is the essence of being human? Is biological humanness the sole criterion? I am sure the Commission for the Protection of Human Subjects has worried over this one all along.

Certainly Dr. Fletcher has been one of the pioneers in the field of biomedical ethics, starting well before the explosion of writing and discussion on the subject in the past decade. This collection of essays embodies some of his major contributions to the field. Read them and worry with them. There are no easy answers.

Thomas H. Hunter, M.D.

Professor of Medicine and Owen
Cheatham Professor of Science, the
University of Virginia

Preface

Everywhere you go these days you run into arguments and headlines about health care and human rights and medical practice. They may be altogether new issues or just old ones in modern dress. I discovered on a recent visit to Minneapolis, for example, that it is the battleground of a debate over whether cardiac pacemakers should shift away from the use of batteries to nuclear fuel. Something like eighty percent of all nuclear-powered implants are manufactured in that city. The issues at stake— questions of cost, patient survival, social hazard, and risk-benefit—drag us deep into the thickets of conscience.

The very notion of "medical ethics" has gone through a radical reconstruction in the past twenty-five years. Until fairly recently it meant a quite moralistic discussion of two things only: medical manners or deportment, and the physician's guild duties. There were paternalistic warnings about not sitting on a patient's bed; not smelling of tobacco or pungent beverages, such as Madeira or even something stronger; how to practice the art of touching, which is what the physician does, but with strict Victorian propriety; and what you owed your professional brothers in the way of respect and discretion. "Remember, Doctor. No bad-mouthing of other doctors. Yours is a fraternity, a guild. Recite the Hippocratic Oath for us," they would say to neophytes, "and then go forth and practice." The American Medical Association Code of 1847 blandly ordered physicians to "unite condescension with authority." Things stayed on that superficial level in medical ethics for another hundred years.

Now see how it has changed. Dr. Howard Brody in 1976 published the first modern textbook on medical ethics written by a physician for medical students.[1] Entitled *Ethical Decisions in Medicine*, it focuses on decision making, not rule following, and it contains not a single word about a physician's etiquette or the guild rules of medical societies. Instead, it deals with open-ended questions like allocating medical resources (not just clinical triage), elective death and proxy powers, quality of life judgments, tissue and organ transplants, guidelines for animal and human experimentation, resuscitation, artificial modes of human reproduction, psychosurgery, fetal interventions, transmission of genetic (not infectious) diseases, and patients' rights. And so on. Medical ethics has graduated into biomedical ethics and biomedical ethics into bioethics— an ethical examination of the life sciences as a whole, in social as well as clinical terms.

In this volume my focus will be on ethics in general, ethics as such, not pinpointed at any one problem but developed within the context of biomedical questions for the sake of concretion. The spectacles we use when we look at our moral problems should be bifocal: one lens to see things up close, one by one, and one lens to see things in the round, pulled together. One without the other is either merely tunnel vision or an abstraction blowing in the wind. We will be taking a hard look at the question which underlies all ethical judgments—How do we decide what is right?—but not as a question philosophically abstracted; it will be explored in the form of quite down-to-earth perplexities.

I am, let me say, a moral philosopher who has managed to escape the toils of nit-picking and logic-chopping. My lot in recent years has fallen in medical education, working with colleagues whose pragmatic temper demands the kind of ethics that seeks practical human benefits as its strongest imperative. In that spirit, let me put the question about how to "do" ethics in terms of a fundamental choice. When we make moral judgments or value choices, decisions as to right and wrong, good and evil, desirable and undesirable, we are, whether we realize it or not, following one or the other of two alternative ethical methods. One strategy is *rule ethics* and the other is *situation ethics*.

Whichever road we go down, as rational human beings we ought to know what we are doing. How we decide what is right (what we "ought" to do) should be conscious with us, and consistent, if we want to preserve our integrity as persons. If physicians, for example, want to nurture the medical arts, they need to understand how they "tick" when they face options or alternative courses of action in which moral values are at stake. When a pediatrician wonders what ought to be done for an irreparably idiotic newborn with a typical congenital anomaly such as duodenal atresia, does he make his moral choice by a rule (Life is always to be preserved) or by the particular clinical situation (In this case to do the surgery would or would not yield a balance of human good over evil)?

In rule ethics we decide what we ought to do *a priori*, according to some predetermined precept or categorical imperative. "You may not terminate this pregnancy because abortion, as such, is wrong." In effect, such rule ethics eliminates what we call conscience—that is, the responsible exercise of moral decision making. If you follow a rule your choice is dictated by the rule. If certain forms or kinds of acts are forbidden in advance of the variables or circumstances of the actual situation, then all decision making has been preempted by the rule. Conscience is irrelevant. The rule decides, and you, the moral agent, have no part to play. (Yours not to reason why, yours but to do and die.)

Situation ethics is the other approach. In their arcane journals philosophers call this *act* ethics. In act or situation ethics the moral agent, the decision maker, judges what is best in the circumstances and in view of foreseeable consequences. This is *a posteriori* rather than *a priori*—after the facts are known, not before. It is, indeed, an ethical strategy consistent with the scientific method. You choose the course of action which offers the greatest (nonmoral) benefit. "Terminating this pregnancy is better than death from cardiac arrest, or (following a positive antenatal diagnosis) to avoid Tay-Sachs disease, or—arguably—simply because the patient is strongly opposed to having a baby." On the other hand, of course, you might by the same method decide, "In this particular case there seems to be no good reason to terminate." It would depend on the case.

Rule ethics is coercive and categorical, not discriminating; situation ethics is open to judgment and seeks the greatest good of the greatest number (for as many as possible of those involved). Rule ethics imposes prefabricated decisions; the moral agent is a null wherever a rule is relevant. In situation ethics what is right sometimes can be wrong at other times, and therefore the moral agent or decision maker is the center of the action.

Rule ethics is deductive; it derives from a rule as the first premise. It says, "Sterilization is wrong and therefore (*ergo*) we may not do a tubal ligation for a patient who does not want to pass on a dominant gene from Huntington's chorea." Situation ethics is inductive, deriving from the facts. It says, "We ought to do whatever is best for the human beings concerned, and in this particular case, on the basis of proportionate good, or what is called gain-loss and risk-benefit, a salpingectomy is called for."

Rule ethics, in short, is a dogmatic or doctrinaire or ideological method of deciding what is right, while situation ethics is relative, flexible, and changeable according to variables. Among modern philosophers and religionists, Immanuel Kant and his categorical imperative and most Catholic (or other) theologians with their divinely ordered "moral law" typify rule ethics; John Stuart Mill and a minority of both Christian and Jewish moralists typify situation ethics. The issue is obviously of great importance for human beings.

Physicians sometimes speak of situation ethics as "clinical" ethics. By training and practice, they appreciate the need of diagnosis and treatment case by case. They are accustomed to judge what is best, not so much according to general rules as according to general principles. Being case-centered and clinically minded, they reject any notion that medicine should be practiced according to moral rules. I would contend that what is good for medicine is good for us all.

Most of us are familiar with the comic strip *Peanuts*, drawn by Charles Schulz. Schulz gives the clue to different kinds of ethical methods. The Lucy type is authoritarian, dogmatic, with punishing taboos and an unbending legalism. Poor Charlie Brown is constantly appalled by her condemnations, but his protesting cry "Good grief!" never moves Lucy. She acts out rule ethics ruthlessly. Little Linus is a subspecies of Lucy; he hugs his moth-eaten blanket to himself—it's his security symbol. All customary or conventional morality gives the ethically timid a place to hide, soft and warm.

Snoopy, in his turn, simply bypasses reality and its complexities. He slips into his fantasies of the Red Baron or the Big Man on Campus, and everything is OK. The easy way out is the way for Snoopy. I maintain, however, that Charlie Brown should be our model. Lucy calls him wishy-washy because he always sees the ambiguities and relativities of moral judgments; unlike her, his main concern is for people, not for categories. The first concern of Charlie Brown, M.D., would be for his patients, not for abstract principles.[2]

The story of abortion and the law is a case in point. For a long time most physicians tabooed abortion because the law did. They legalistically refused to terminate pregnancies except for the most serious medical indications and even then only through the so-called T.A. (therapeutic abortion) committees. For all other cases they would turn to one scapegoat physician in the community; their clandestine referrals achieved what they were afraid to do. Finally the Supreme Court in *Roe* v. *Wade* cut through the rule morality of state laws and freed physicians to do what they were willing all along to do, for both humanistic and medical reasons. It took the top justices of the land to demonstrate more human-ity and flexibility than the medical profession could muster.

The fundamental ethical question is whether we are to live and act by rules or by reason. What I have tried to say in this book is that it is wiser to be guided by moral principles than by moral rules, and that this wisdom is specially appropriate to the medical sciences and medical arts.

Long ago in classical Greece, medicine was done according to the Dogmatist cults as exemplified by Empedocles and Pythagoras; it was based on metaphysics and religion. Under the leadership of Hippocrates, they broke away and based their medicine on empirical rather than metaphysical foundations. Ethics could learn a valuable lesson from this. Unfortunately, Empedocles and Pythagoras are still with us in the form of conscience, and will continue to reign there as long as we practice rule ethics.

Modern medicine got its start when it shifted away from Galen's reliance on rules and tried and true remedies, going instead to Paracelsus and his teaching that experience is more important than tradition. This insight is the very heart of situation ethics. The spirit of modern medicine is the best model for ethics, not only medicine's ethics, but all ethics.

1. Howard Brody, *Ethical Decisions in Medicine* (Boston: Little Brown and Company, 1976).

2. This amusing typology was suggested by C. R. Woodruff, "Pastoral Considerations in Abortion and Sterilization," *Pastoral Psychology* 24 (Fall, 1975) 288, 40-51.

One

Humanness

We are constantly seeing lists, which grow longer all the time, of ethical questions in biomedical research and clinical practice. What ought we to do, or not do, about such things as truthtelling in medical diagnosis, sterilization, transplants and implants, intensive care and "crash" treatments, defective newborns and high-risk pregnancies, *in vitro* fertilizations in embryology, triage decisions about things like complicated hepatic coma, abortions, and genetic therapy and design proposals. We should include, also, behavior control by psychosurgery or chemotherapy, positive and negative euthanasia, cyborg amplifications, transsexual surgery, selection procedures for hemodialysis and other scarcity allocations, artificial insemination and inovulation, refusals of consent to indicated treatment, "ghost" surgery and medical care, the non-medicinal use of drugs, clinical experiments, fetologic interventions. The list is long and, as I say, growing.

As Robert Morison has pointed out,[1] "There are several reasons for believing that we can no longer keep our system of morality and our system of scientific expertise in separate water-tight compartments. Perhaps most important is the fact that science, and especially biological science, has produced evidence to reinforce some ancient exhortations and weaken the hold of others, and has invented, or at least called attention to the significance of, an entirely new range of good and bad behavior."

Physicians and biologists are notoriously conservative people, but by their "intranaut" research into the chemical depths of men they have precipitated an ethical and social revolution far more portentous than the astronauts' moon-walks and rock collecting. Now, with man's new control over man himself, by the new genetics, birth technologies, and life-support systems—now, what ought we to be doing and not doing, and how do we understand this "man" who makes and remakes men?

Morally speaking, how simple medicine and medical education were sixty years ago, i.e., up to the time that the random patient with the random complaint had even a 50-50 chance of being helped by the random physician. As medicine's achievements proliferate, and as its control of life, health, and death increases, the frequency, complexity, and subtlety of its decision making also necessarily increase. And the part played by values in the decisional mix therefore increases. The essence of biomedical decision making can be put this way: What, of what can be done, should be done; what of what should be done can we afford; and what of what we can afford are we prepared to pay?

Cost-benefit and trade-off judgments loom larger all the time, and thornier. If medicine is, as we commonly believe, for the good of human beings, then it follows, does it not, that physicians had better not only have some sense of value priorities but, more particularly, some idea of who or what human beings are—those for whose sake they make their decisions. Words like "humane" and "humanistic" and claims that this or that violates "the very nature of man" will be murky semantic swamps until this task of analysing and explicating medicine's concept of man is tackled with at least some measure of agreed success.

Some ethicists have expressed a doubt that the "humanhood inventory" can succeed. They may prove to be right, but the evidence is not in and will not be in until far more work has been done on it biologically, philosophically, and theologically—far more than anything done to date. Others speak of it as "the crucial question." In any case, unfortunately, our inherited classical accounts of "man" have been far too metaphysically or religiously based on discredited ontogenies and ontologies, both, although biomedical re-examination may conceivably revalidate or reinforce at least some features of the ancient and medieval notions of the *humanum*.

Abortion provides a clinical context in which we can see the need of a consensual answer to the question, What is a human being? and our serious lack of one. There are other medical situations in which it is equally critical, however. I recall the decision making of a California prison's medical staff when confronted by a nonpsychotic prisoner's request for a prefrontal lobotomy. He had been imprisoned for committing murder in a rage, then murdered a fellow inmate—and finally almost killed a prison guard. What would he be like after the operation? What was risked? Could it be justified? Quality-of-life analyses obviously depend on some presuppositions about human biology and social welfare, but those who make their moral judgments by a quality-of-life ethics will, especially, need a list of criteria for humanness to supply the parameters of quality judgments and selections. The American Association for the Advancement of Science at its 1971 meeting began an interesting interdisciplinary inquiry, hoping to construct a quality-of-life index, but their task seems impossible without a profile of humanness— if "quality of life" is quality for the sake of human beings, as I presume it is.

In the same way, I think, the question transcends or prescinds from the issue as between theism, which puts God at the center of its outlook, and humanism, which puts man at the center. Whether we believe with Protagoras that men are the measure of things, or with the Bible, that God is, it behooves us to decide what we are talking about, to have a responsible and intelligible meaning for *man*. And, if possible, a meaning shared with others.

In my opinion, the task of manhood inventory should be carried out from the humanistic perspective rather than a theistic one. We should deliberately and consciously omit any claim to "knowing God's will"— claiming nothing beyond the conviction that any God worth believing in intends the highest possible well-being for human beings, or what the Bible calls love. In short, we should assume that there can be no practical difference in the ethical judgments of humanistically and theologically oriented moral agents. Our guideline, then, would be what is humane and rational, not what is revealed or authoritarian.

This is a meta-ethical or pre-ethical question which needs careful discussion. I may be in error here, although I don't think I am. If I am, then how—exactly, in operational terms—does it make a difference in our profile of man's traits if we do or do not posit faith in God? Nearly all of what little postmedieval inquiry there has been into this question has been carried out without using God-talk, by physical and cultural anthropology, psychology, and biology. See, for example, the studies by Sherrington, Comfort, Dubos, Dobzhansky, and the Rathbones.[2]

We all know the dangers of reductionism, i.e., the tendency to explain personality in terms of physiology, physiology in terms of metabolism, metabolism in terms of biochemistry, biochemistry in terms of chemistry, chemistry in terms of molecules, and molecules in terms of atoms, so that since the behavior of atoms is notoriously random, you end up with a question mark! Nevertheless, I would want to defend old Thomas Huxley's point made a hundred years ago, defending Darwin from the charge of godlessness; using a physical model to understand nature, including man, does not make us materialists or atheists any more than eating food or wearing clothes do.

We have, therefore, only a starting point in the answer of an editor of a medical journal to the question What is Man? "He is the only animal that can smile, I think Darwin said, but I have seen other primates smile, and my poodle sometimes seems to smile; and all dogs wag their tails, which is their way of smiling. He is the only animal that needs clothes and wears clothes. He has more heartbeats per lifetime than other animals. He has an opposable thumb. He walks erect on his lower extremities. He cleans himself after defecating. He marries, but cardinals, redbirds, that is, do too. He is the only animal capable of the face to face coital position. He speaks. He prays."

The editor continues: "He sometimes cuts his hair and shaves his beard, and she shaves her legs and axillae. He has no tail. He is omnivorous, but systematically; he grows plants and raises other animals to eat. He bathes. He thinks. He pollutes, but other animals do, too. He kills, and not for food. He is the only animal that takes drugs. And he gets drunk. He is the only animal without zero population growth. And he writes."[3]

By the phrase *nature of man* I would hope we do not mean *human nature*. The phrase *nature of man* is acceptable because it calls for a description, which is our task in meta-ethics. *Human nature* however, connotes a substantive and even fixed nature, as something "given in the nature of things," *de rerum natura*, an idea which may be seen classically in the old natural law tradition of prescientific reasoning. As recently as 1924, we find T. E. Hulme saying, "Man is an extraordinarily fixed and limited animal whose nature is absolutely constant."[4] Less radical versions assign a kind of residual and unchanging core of human being. Contrasted to this is the opinion of René Dubos that man "has the privilege and responsibility of shaping his self and his future."[5] In our investigation I would range myself with Ortega y Gasset's argument that man has no nature, only a history,[6] and with Ashley Montagu's observation[7] that babies are not born with human nature, but only with more or less capacity to become human. To some people in medical education this will seem a very abstruse issue, but such thinking is superficial.

Another point of prolegomena is that our analysis of the question, What is a man? needs to be converted in its form to, What is a person? A glance at arguments about the ethics of abortion and euthanasia is enough to make my reasons clear. Sometimes discussants say that whether it is right or not to terminate a pregnancy depends on whether an embryo or fetus is a human life. But that is not the critical question any more. Of course it is alive. Cell division goes forward from fertilization. And of course it is human, since any biologist could quickly identify even a blastula as of the species *Homo sapiens*—not as a monkey's or a rabbit's. No: the question is not whether it is a life or even whether it is a human life. The question is whether we may assign personal status to fetal life—the status that is usually meant when people speak of "a truly human being."

Adrian Kantrowitz, the eminent brain surgeon, spoke once of "reverence for life" as the ethics of medicine. But the issue, then, is around reverence, how we revere life. Does it mean concern for life-as-such (a mystical outlook)? Nobody in his right mind regards life as sacrosanct. Then is it concern for the quality of life (a critical outlook)? And is it just life we revere, or is it human life? Some would condemn taking human life—radical pacifists, for example, and opponents of capital punishment, although some of them would nevertheless justify homicide in self-defense. But is it even human life, actually, that medical ethics is concerned with, or personal life? When we quote the Socratic maxim, Know thyself, what is the self, what is the person, what is the man?

Defective fetuses, defective newborns, moribund patients—all of these are human lives. Some physicians would "sacrifice" such human lives sometimes, others would not. But do they understand the import of their policy? If there is any ground at all, ethically, as I would contend there is, for allowing or hastening the end of such lives, it must be on a qualitative ground, that such human lives are subpersonal. What is critical is personal status, not merely human status. This is why the law does not allow that a fetus is a person.

I am not entering here into the issue whether abortion and euthanasia are defensible. (I will deal at length with these questions later.) Here I am only illustrating the fundamental importance of the question about the nature of man. A "man," I would want to contend, is not just human, he is a person. There are, as physicians know so well, some human beings who either will never become, or have ceased to be, persons.

It is not what is natural but what is personal which has the first-order value in ethics. Sir Peter Medawar states it succinctly: "It is a profound truth...that nature does not know best; that genetical evolution, if we choose to look at it liverishly instead of with fatuous good humor, is a story of waste, makeshift, compromise, and blunder."[8]

Mark Twain complained that people are always talking about the weather but they never do anything about it. The same is true of humanhood criteria. In biomedical ethics writers constantly say that we need to explicate humanness or humaneness, what it means to be a truly human being, but they never follow their admission of the need with an actual inventory or profile, no matter how tentatively offered. Yet this is what must be done, or at least attempted.

Synthetic concepts such as human and man and person require operational terms, spelling out the which and what and when. Only in that way can we get down to cases—to normative decisions. There are always some people who prefer to be visceral and affective in their moral choices, with no desire to have any rationale for what they do. But ethics is precisely the business of rational, critical reflection (encephalic and not merely visceral) about the problems of the moral agent—in biology and medicine as much as in law, government, education, or anything else.

To that end, then, for the purposes of biomedical ethics, I now turn to a *profile of man* in concrete and discrete terms. As only one man's reflection on man, it will no doubt invite adding and subtracting by others, but this is the road to be followed if we mean business. As a dog is said to worry a bone, let me worry out loud and on paper, hoping for some agreement and, at the least, consideration. There is time only to itemize the inventory, not to enlarge upon it, but I have fifteen positive propositions and five negative propositions. Let me set them out, in no rank order at all, and as hardly more than a list of criteria or indicators, by simple title.

1. Minimum intelligence

Any individual of the species *Homo sapiens* who falls below an I.Q. grade of 40 in a standard Stanford-Binet test, amplified if you like by other tests, is questionably a person; below the mark of 20, not a person. *Homo* is indeed *sapiens*, in order to be *Homo*. The *ratio*, in another turn of speech, is what makes a person of the *vita*. Mere biological life, before minimal intelligence is achieved or after it is lost irretrievably, is without personal status. This has bearing, obviously, on decision making in gynecology, obstetrics, and pediatrics, as well as in general surgery and medicine.

2. Self-awareness

Self-consciousness, as we know, is the quality we watch developing in a baby; we watch it with fascination and glee. Its essential role in personality development is a basic datum of psychology. Its existence or function in animals at or below the primate level is debatable. It is clearly absent in the lower vertebrates, as well as in the nonvertebrates. In psychotherapy non-self-awareness is pathological; in medicine, unconsciousness when it is incorrigible at once poses quality-of-life judgments—for example, in neurosurgical cases of irreversible damage to the brain cortex.

3. Self-control

If an individual is not only not controllable by others (unless by force) but not controllable by the individual himself or herself, a low level of life is reached about on a par with that of a paramecium. If the condition cannot be rectified medically, so that means-ends behavior is out of the question, the individual is not a person—not ethically, and certainly not in the eyes of the law—just as a fetus is not legally a person.

4. A sense of time

Time consciousness. By this is meant clock time or *chronos*, not timeliness or *kairos*, i.e., not the "fullness of time" or the pregnant moment (remember Paul Tillich?). A sense, that is, of the passage of time. Dr. Thomas Hunter, a colleague of mine and Professor of Medicine at the University of Virginia, remarked recently, "Life is the allocation of time." We can disagree legitimately about how relatively important this indicator is, but it is hard to understand why anybody would minimize it or eliminate it as a trait of humanness.

5. A sense of futurity

How "truly human" is any man who cannot realize there is a time yet to come as well as the present? Subhuman animals do not look forward in time; they live only on what we might call visceral strivings, appetites. Philosophical anthropologies (one recalls that of William Temple, the Archbishop of Canterbury, for instance) commonly emphasize purposiveness as a key to humanness. Chesterton once remarked that we would never ask a puppy what manner of dog it wanted to be when it grows up. The assertion here is that men are typically teleological, although certainly not eschatological. For the latter sense of futurity, the eschatological outlook, and its ethical input, see Ramsey[9], who reasons that we ought not to aim teleologically at what is good (a consequentialist ethics) but act according to whatever we may believe about the "eschaton," or man's eternal and supernatural destiny.

6. A sense of the past

Memory. Unlike other animals, men as a species have reached a unique

level of neurologic development, particularly in the cerebrum and especially its neocortex. They are linked to the past by conscious recall—not
only, as with subhuman animals, by conditioning and the reactivation of
emotions (reactivated, that is, externally rather than autonomously). It is
this trait, in particular, that makes man, alone among all species, a
cultural instead of an instinctive creature. An existentialist focus on
"nowness" truncates the nature of man.

7. The capability to relate to others

Interpersonal relationships, of the sexual-romantic and friendship
kind, are of the greatest importance for the fulness of what we idealize as
being truly personal. Medical piety in the past has always held its professional ethics to be only a one-to-one, physician-patient obligation.
However, there are also the more diffuse and comprehensive social
relations of our vocational, economic, and political life. Aristotle's characterization of man as a social animal, *zoon politikon*, must surely figure
prominently in the inventory. It is true that even insects live in social
systems, but the cohesion of all subhuman societies is based on instinct.
Man's society is based on culture—that is, on a conscious knowledge of
the system and on the exercise in some real measure of either consent or
opposition.

8. Concern for others

Some people may be skeptical about our capacity to care about others
(what in Christian ethics is often distinguished from romance and friendship as "neighbor love" or "neighbor concern"). The extent to which
this capacity is actually in play is debatable. But whether concern for
others is disinterested or inspired by enlightened self-interest, it seems
plain that a conscious extra-ego orientation is a trait of the species; the
absence of this ambience is a clinical indication of psychopathology.

9. Communication

Utter alienation or disconnection from others, if it is irreparable, is
de-humanization. This is not so much a matter of not being disposed to
receive and send "messages" as of the inability to do so. This criterion
comes into question in patients who cannot hear, speak, feel, or see
others. It may come about as a result of mental or physical trauma,
infection, genetic or congenital disorder, or from psychological causes.
Completely and finally isolated individuals are subpersonal. The prob-

lem is perhaps most familiar in terminal illnesses and the clinical decision making required.

10. Control of existence

It is of the nature of man that he is not helplessly subject to the blind workings of physical or physiological nature. He has only finite knowledge, freedom, and initiative, but what he has of it is real and effective. Invincible ignorance and total helplessness are the antithesis of humanness, and to the degree that a man lacks control he is not responsible, and to be irresponsible is to be subpersonal. This item in the agenda applies directly, for example, in psychiatric medicine, especially to severe cases of toxic and degenerative psychosis.

11. Curiosity

To be without affect, sunk in *anomie*, is to be not a person. Indifference is inhuman. Man is a learner and a knower as well as a tool maker and user. This raises a question, therefore, about demands to stop some kinds of biomedical inquiry. For example, an AMA committee recently imposed a ban on *in vitro* fertilization and embryo transplants on the ground that they are dangerous. But dangerous ignorance is more dangerous than dangerous knowledge. It is dehumanizing to impose a moratorium on research. No doubt this issue arises, or will arise, in many other phases of medical education and practice.

12. Change and changeability

To the extent that an individual is unchangeable or opposed to change, he denies the creativity of personal beings. It means not only the fact of biological and physiological change, which goes on as a condition of life, but the capacity and disposition for changing one's mind and conduct as well. Biologically, human beings are developmental: birth, life, health, and death are processes, not events, and are to be understood progressively, not episodically. All human existence is on a continuum, a matter of becoming. In this perspective, are we to regard potentials *als ob*, as if they were actual? I think not. The question arises prominently in abortion ethics.

13. Balance of rationality and feeling

To be "truly human," to be a wholesome person, one cannot be either Apollonian or Dionysian. As human beings we are not coldly rational or cerebral, nor are we merely creatures of feeling and intuition. It is a matter of being both, in different combinations from one individual to another. To be one rather than the other is to distort the *humanum*.

14. Idiosyncrasy

The human being is idiomorphous, a distinctive individual. As Helmut Schoeck has shown,[10] even the function of envy in human behavior is entirely consistent with idiosyncrasy. To be a person is to have an identity, to be recognizable and callable by name. It is this criterion which lies behind the fear that to replicate individuals by so-called cloning would be to make carbon copies of the parent source and thus dehumanize the clone by denying it its individuality. One or two writers have even spoken of a "right" to a "unique genotype," and while such talk is ethically and scientifically questionable, it nonetheless reflects a legitimate notion of something essential to an authentic person.

15. Neocortical function

In a way, this is the cardinal indicator, the one all the others are hinged upon. Before cerebration is in play, or with its end, in the absence of the synthesizing function of the cerebral cortex, the person is nonexistent. Such individuals are objects but not subjects. This is so no matter how many other spontaneous or artificially supported functions persist in the heart, lungs, neurologic and vascular systems. Such noncerebral processes are not personal. Like the Harvard Medical School's *ad hoc* committee report on "brain death," some state statutes require the absence of brain function. So do the guidelines for the legal determination of death recently adopted by the Italian Council of Ministers. But what is definitive in determining death is the loss of cerebration, not just of any or all brain function. Personal reality depends on cerebration and to be dead "humanly" speaking is to be excerebral, no matter how long the body remains alive.

The five negative points I have can be put even more briefly than the fifteen positive ones, although I am inclined to believe that they merit just as much critical scrutiny and elaboration.

1. Man is not non- or anti-artificial

Men are characterized by technique, and for a human being to oppose technology is self-hatred. We are often confused on this score, attitudinally. A "test tube baby," for example, although conceived and gestated *ex corpo*, would nonetheless be humanly reproduced and of human value. A baby made artificially, by deliberate and careful contrivance, would be more human than one resulting from sexual roulette—the reproductive mode of the subhuman species.

2. Man is not essentially parental

People can be fully personal without reproducing, as the religious vows of nuns, monks, and celibate priests of the past have asserted, as the law has implied by refusing to annul marriages because of sterility, and as we see in the ethos reversal of contemporary family and population control—and, more militantly, in the nonparental rhetoric of women's liberation and a growing rejection of the "baby trap."

3. Man is not essentially sexual

Sexuality, a broader and deeper phenomenon than sex, is of the fullness but not of the essence of man. It is not even necessary to human species survival. I will not try here to indicate the psychological entailments of this negative proposition, but it is biologically apparent when we look at such nonsexual reproduction as cloning from somatic cells and parthenogenetic reproduction by both androgenesis and gynogenesis. What light does this biology throw on the nature of man? what does a personistic view of man say about the ethics of such biology? (N.B. I do not refer here to personalism, which has more metaphysical freight than many of us want to carry.)

4. Man is not a bundle of rights

The notion of a human nature has served as a conceptual bucket to contain "human rights" and certain other given things, like "original sin" and "the sense of oughtness" and "conscience." The idea behind this is that such things are objective, pre-existent phenomena, not contingent on biological or social relativities. People sometimes speak of rights to live, to die, to be healthy, to reproduce, and so on, as if they were absolute, eternal, intrinsic. But as the law makes plain, all rights are imperfect and may be set aside if human need requires it. We shall have to think through the relation of rights and needs, as it bears on clinical medicine's decision-making problems, as well as society's problems of health care delivery. One example: What is the "humane" policy if we should reach the point (I think we will) of deciding for or against compulsory birth control? Or, how are we to relate rights and needs if, to take only one example, an ethnic group protests against mass screening for sickle cell anemia? Or if after genetic counseling, a couple elects to proceed with a predictably degenerate pregnancy?

5. Man is not a worshipper

Faith in supernatural realities and attempts to be in direct association with them are choices some human beings make and others do not. Mystique is not essential to being truly a person. Like sexuality, it may arguably be of the fullness of humanness but it is not of the essence. This negative proposition is required by our basic guideline, the premise that a workable biomedical ethics is humanistic, whatever reasons we may have for putting human well-being at the center of concern.

These are the criteria, but how are we to go about testing them? And how are we to compare and combine the results of our criticism? How are we to rank-order or give priority to the items in our man-hood profile? Which are only optimal, what are essential? What are the applications of these or other indicators to the normative decisions of biologists and physicians? In my own list, here, which factors can be eliminated, in whole or in part, without lowering individuals and patients below the personal line? I trust that by this time it is plain that I do not claim to have produced the pure gospel of humanness. I remain open to correction.

The nature of man question is of such depth and sensitivity that it is bound to raise controversy, and our task is to welcome the controversy but try to reduce it through analysis and synthesis. Said Heraclitus: "Opposition brings concord. Out of discord comes the fairest harmony. It is by disease that health is pleasant; by evil that good is pleasant; by hunger, satiety; by weariness, rest."[11]

I rather suspect that we are more apt to find good answers inductively and empirically, from medical science and the clinicians, than by the necessarily syllogistic reasoning of the humanities, which proceeds deductively from abstract premises. Syllogisms always contain their conclusions in their major or first premises. Divorced from the laboratory and the hospital, talk about what it means to be human could easily become inhumane.

1. Robert Morison, *Science* 155 (1967) 431.

2. Alex Comfort, *The Nature of Human Nature* (New York: Harper & Row, 1966). Theodosius Dobzhansky, *Heredity and the Nature of Man,* (New York: Harcourt, Brace & World, 1964). Rene Dubos, *Man Adapting,* (New Haven: Yale University Press, 1965). F. S. Rathbone and E. T. Rathbone, *Health and Human Values* (New York: McGraw-Hill, Inc., 1971). C. S. Sherrington, *Man on His Nature* (New York: The Macmillan Company, 1941).

3. Frederick Cole, *Nebraska State Medical Journal* 56 (1971) 211.

4. T. E. Hulme, *Speculation: Essays on Humanism and the Philosophy of Art* (New York: Harcourt & Brace, 1946), 11.

5. René Dubos, *So Human an Animal* (New York: Charles Scribner's Sons, 1968) 106.

6. José Ortega y Gasset, *Man and People,* trans. W. R. Trask (New York: W. W. Norton and Company, 1957).

7. Ashley Montagu, *Sex, Man and Society* (New York: G. P. Putnam's Sons, 1969).

8. Peter B. Medawar, *The Future of Man* (London: Methuen and Company, 1960), 100.

9. Paul Ramsey, *Fabricated Man: The Ethics of Genetic Control* (New Haven: Yale University Press, 1970), 30.

10. Helmut Schoeck, *Envy: A Theory of Social Behavior* (New York: Harcourt, Brace & World, 1966).

11. Heraclitus of Ephesus, *The Cosmic Fragments,* ed. G. S. Kirk (Cambridge: Cambridge University Press, 1954), 98-99.

Two

Happiness

Only by deciding what we believe it means to be human, in terms such as I have outlined, can we look equally closely at what it means to be happy.

The point at issue was dramatized in a symposium I once took part in at a grand rounds in the Texas Medical Center in Houston. The panelists were wrestling with the moral problem of whether pediatricians may ever end a defective newborn's life and, if so, for what reasons. The panel was widely diversified: it included clinicians, scientists, philosophers, theologizers, lawyers—the whole gamut of experience and opinion.

I contended that any decision to end, sustain, or repair the life of a seriously diseased or deformed infant would be right or wrong only relatively and that in each case the decision would have to be made on the basis of the facts in the particular case or situation. That is, such decisions should be clinical, not ideological. But being pressed (reasonably enough) for a definition of what it is to be truly human, I proposed that the *sine qua non*—the indispensable trait or criterion—is mind, what we call cerebration and what our forebears called mentation.

Besides cerebration there are most assuredly other important optimal traits (self-awareness, communicativeness, purposiveness, and so on), but it is still true that the essential, minimal quality of any truly human individual is the ability to be reflective, to carry out those synthesizing and voluntary functions of the cerebral cortex that we call thinking. Other things besides cerebration, yes; but without that one trait all the others would at most add up to subhuman. To the ears of those whom

William James called "the tender-minded," it sounded, I am sure, like a hard or coldly rationalistic definition.

One doctor present had this retort: "I work in a program for retarded children. In our institution we have a little boy three years old. His IQ is practically zero. Still and all, the child is happy. He is happy all the time. He responds warmly and affectionately to every attention and shows a capacity for joy that any of us might envy. I tell you, you could not possibly look at that little boy and then say he isn't a human being."

What was the doctor saying? It seems plain enough. She was saying that euphoria is what constitutes humanhood, that we are real people or persons if we have a feeling of happiness or well-being, regardless of whether we have any capacity for thought and reason. This contrasts radically with the traditional view of the European Judeo-Christian world, where it has always been held that the *ratio*, or reason, establishes the *humanum* and that man's capacity to transcend merely instinctual responses to stimuli by the workings of his mind is what makes him superior to all other species of creatures (even though he may still be "lower than the angels"). The nub of the matter, then, is that we cannot sing hosannas to happiness or preach a gospel of joy unless and until we say what kind of happiness or joy we mean.

Webster's dictionary defines euphoria as "a feeling of well-being or elation; especially: one that is groundless, disproportionate to its cause, or inappropriate to one's own life situation." Those who are euphoric, in other words, are cut off from reality. If I were ever unfortunate enough to get cut off from reality—from what psychiatrists call the "reality situation"—and it was only temporary, I would, I suppose, want to be in a state of euphoria rather than melancholia. If, in a far more ominous case, my trouble were a permanent and incurable psychosis, I would nonetheless still be a human being because I had a mind, no matter how disordered. But to be mindless, unable to think, even falsely and foolishly, would be subhuman or nonhuman, no matter how "good" I might feel, no matter whether I were only seven hours old or a full seven decades.

Since the notion of culpability or blameworthiness first was appreciated by humankind, law and ethics have made it plain that civilized people believe that the lack or loss of reason excuses wrongdoers. In the forum of conscience we are not responsible and therefore not answerable if and when we do not know or cannot understand the consequences of what we do; the ability to think consequentially is the basis of moral competence. Both law and morality assume that, without sufficient mind to reason about the effects of what we do, we are not to be blamed. Such is the case with children and morons and imbeciles. Further than this, even mature and competent persons may be exculpated in cases of great emotional stress, temporary insanity, inadvertence, or invincible ignorance. Their excuse is simply that they could not think.

Idiots, however, are another matter. They are not, never were, and never will be in any degree responsible. Idiots, that is to say, are not human. The problem they pose is not lack of sufficient mind, but of any mind at all. No matter how euphoric their behavior might be, they are outside the pale of human integrity. Indeed, sustained and "plateau" euphoria is itself *prima facie* clinical evidence of mindlessness.

Euphoria is, of course, not a feature of all idiocy. There are non-cerebral newborns who show no clinical signs of pleasure-affect at all. And by the same token, some ex-cerebral patients may be entirely without pleasure feelings. Examples would be children whose neocortex has been suffocated (anoxia) in accidents at play and auto accident victims or attempted suicides whose massive brain injuries leave all spontaneous activities of their brain stems and body organs intact and functioning, yet whose mental functions are gone irrecoverably. Such patients are no longer human beings; the body is still there breathing and digesting and eliminating, but the person is gone.

Creative joy and happiness are not euphoria but intelligent pleasure. The operative word is intelligent. And to be a human being it is essential, not just optimal or desirable, that an individual have the intelligence to control and select his pleasures. Mindless pleasure is seen in the idiot's euphoria, just as it may be seen in the compulsive pleasure-hunger of the Norway rat. When an electrode is implanted in the limbic area of its brain, or what Olds called "the rivers of reward," the rat, by pressing a lever, can experience "pure" pleasure and always does so to the complete neglect of food, water, sex, and sleep—keeping it up until stopped by utter exhaustion. If the rat is "happy," it is arguably not having true rodent happiness—and the idiot certainly is not having human happiness.

I have no wish to be overly rationalistic or to appear like a cold-blooded intellectual who wants minds that merely work like computers. On the contrary, I have argued that a full and rich humanness (the *bene esse* of being human) calls for a creative and happy balance of the Apollonian and Dionysian principles—a sensitive commixture of mind and feeling. If the cerebral and the visceral fail to work together, humanity is threatened. Mind without emotion is impoverished; emotion without mind is squalid. But always and necessarily, mind, not emotion, is the essence. They make a beautiful partnership, but only if brains are boss.

When William James distinguished the "tender" and the "tough" minded—those in whom feeling is uppermost and those in whom reason is uppermost—he did not forget to explain that the qualities have to go together, each to the other's profit. In the famous first chapter of *Pragmatism* he explained why they need each other, although this part of his classic treatise is too often ignored. The point is, he left no doubt that without rigorous reason, when only the "tender" side is at work, there is "nobody home in the upper story."

In the history of ideas we can trace the sad waste of time and effort that follows when we slide into the semantic swamp, when we confuse terms or lose the meaning of some of our most familiar words. The tyranny of words, as Stuart Chase called it, has always plagued our discussions of happiness.

Socrates, in the Protagoras dialogue, was the first to lay out the theory for a humanist ethics based on happiness or human utility. From Plato and Aristotle down to the modern utilitarians there has been a general agreement among thoughtful people that happiness is the highest good. But true as it is that the proposition is ancient and widely upheld, what a semantic snare and delusion the statement always was and is.

Homer and Herodotus understood happiness or pleasure to be basically physical satisfaction, as the Cyrenaics did, but others, like the Epicureans, thought of happiness as rather more of a moral and intellectual satisfaction. So-called hedonists (*heidonei* is the Greek word for pleasure) disagreed among themselves: some thought of pleasure as physical, others as mental. (For example, Epicurus, founder of the movement named for him, urged celibacy as a necessary condition for seeking the good things of true pleasure. This was, of course, a nonissue, an unreal either-or, but it serves to show the semantic confusion of words like "happiness," "joy," "pleasure," "gratification," and "satisfaction.")

When Aristotle and Plato talked about happiness or eudaemonia (literally "good spirits," but usually translated "well-being"), they meant happiness based on more than pleasurable sensations. Aristotle said that happiness is the harmonious fulfillment of our natural desires (the Golden Mean). Plato, in his Socratic period, distinguished between noble and base pleasures, meaning in effect, as we have been saying, that truly human pleasures are intelligent—not just mindless sensation, not just full bellies and orgasms. Let us have full bellies and better orgasms, by all means, but not as ends in themselves. They do not establish our humanness. After all, every one of our biological functions, including sex and gestation, is shared with all the other mammals, from the primates down.

Later, when he was influenced by the Pythagoreans, especially Timaeus, Plato condemned physical pleasure as such and turned to a kind of body rejection, writing nonsense about the "inferior soul" below the neck. This negation of pleasure was followed by St. Augustine, who reinterpreted happiness (*beatitas*) ascetically, to exclude physical satisfactions, thus setting a theological pattern for the Christian denial of the body and for antisexual attitudes. (This dualism of the physical and the spiritual has been, as we now commonly see, a canker at the heart of the Christian heritage.)

Wherever people stand on the spectrum of defining pleasure, from animal sensations to rarified intellectual achievements, they all declare happiness to be the highest good. Words are treacherous when their reach is too broad to discriminate. Happiness runs this risk; it can be claimed for rats with limbic electrodes or for victims of nymphomania or satyriasis (compulsive sexual behavior) or for architects with a passionate vocational preoccupation or for a dried-up monk with his mystique in a monastic cell or for the composer of a new symphony. What counts in happiness is whether its pleasures have a rational function. That is to say, happiness is authentically human only if its satisfactions are free, selective, and purposive—in short, mentally controlled.

The utilitarians today (I count myself among them) hold that a moral agent's business is to maximize the good, which they define as happiness. As Mill said, the foundation of values and morals is "Utility, or the Greatest Happiness Principle." Whatever is useful for increasing human happiness is good; whatever reduces human happiness is evil. But the hoary old questions still nag us for an answer: Are we to understand happiness as sensational (midbrain) or rational (cortex)? Utilitarians have a distinction between the hedonists and the nonhedonists—the former being the Cyrenaic sensationalists and the latter the Epicurean rationalists.

John Stuart Mill made a strong case for what I have described as pleasure as a rational function. Jeremy Bentham, on the other hand, said that playing pushpin is as pleasurable for some as poetry is for others, and therefore they are equally good. It is obvious that Bentham personally shared Mill's preference for mathematics and poetry over pushpin and black stout, but by equating both kinds of happiness, he reduced happiness to what the Greeks called a panchreston, an idea that explained everything in general but nothing in particular.

The thrust of this essay is to challenge Bentham's concept of happiness, his notion that the sensate is equal to the rational, that feeling equals mind. To reduce happiness to physical pleasure is ultimately antihumanistic. What counts if happiness is to be human is whether its constitutent satisfactions are rational. The principle is: Happiness is a function of reason.

Neither Apollo nor Dionysus is an irrational or mindless model for man. It is true that the Apollonian spirit loves logic and analysis and critical reason and knowledge, but it also keeps a generous place in its scheme of things for values, aesthetic needs, and imagination. When it ignores them it suffers impoverishment in consequence. On the other side, the Dionysian spirit or ethos puts its premium on human feelings and strivings; yet only when it runs amok—away from rational limits—does it allow sensitivity of feeling to degenerate into "pure" feeling, thus falsifying humanhood. Poets are quite commonly addicted to puzzles and game problems, as we all know, and mathematicians are noted for their love of music.

Western man has never seriously entertained the belief, once peddled by disciples of the Iranian Zoroaster, that flesh and feeling are evil, mind and spirit are good. This antihedonism crept into the Christian Church through the Manichaeans and Augustine. Augustine formally condemned it as a heresy but nevertheless built it into his theology, teaching that the only excuse for sex was that it made babies with souls, which needed the church to save them. But the cankerous taboo never really caught on except with a few true believers. Nor will very many ever accept its opposite form, that of the counter-culture kids, who express it as a revolt against reason, in vacant jungle music, in the "mind-blowing" ecstasy of Jesus freaks and the Indian-guru followers, or by deliberately "going out of their gourds" on drugs.

Biochemists at the University of Michigan have used submammalian test animals to learn how we can turn down the biological thermostat controlling our body temperature. The lower it goes, the slower the aging process, short of some minimum survival level. Results show that to push the body's temperature down from 98.6 to about 86 degrees would add about twenty years to our lives, not only increasing our longevity but also reducing the incidence of some of the main man-killers—vascular disease, cancer, and heart trouble. Next will come work on mammals, than on human subjects.

Now, suppose this reduction of body heat is found to be a threat to the life of the emotions, or at least to the intensity of our feelings, thus throwing the weight of our lives biologically against the Dionysian principle and in favor of the Apollonian. Where is the break-off point? Food, sex, and shelter are hardly enough in themselves to provide the intellect with the affect needed for a mature and perceptive quality of life and mind. When would we begin paying too much for the sake of more years and better health? At what point would we decide we prefer risking the possibility of cancer and cardiac failure to any further loss of our subjective and emotive powers? Here is a trade-off or cost-benefit problem worthy of this miraculous age of ours. And it is not a merely academic or science-fiction question.

The age-old issue still confronts us. To use a traditional and familiar way of putting it, although we hold happiness to be the highest good, which kind of happiness do we want? Socrates' happiness or a pig's? Or, a harder question: Which is good, Socrates unhappy, or his pig happy?

Three

Goodness

In a very real way humanness and happiness depend in their turn on goodness or quality. Quality in things and deeds, both. These are ethical notions, value judgments. You might say that ethics is choosing between competing values, which means we *all* "do" ethics. What, then, do we mean when we say something is *good*? How should be go about choosing options in life? How does *being good* relate to doing what is right?

The upshot of what follows here will be that virtue is only a predicate, in the sense of an attribution of a certain quality to a moral act or a moral agent—not in any way a property of or in it. More succinctly, virtue is nominal, not real; it is extrinsic to acts and agents, not intrinsic. In short, virtue lies in the utility that an act *happens* to have in a particular situation, for the sake of or attainment of one value or another. (An extension of this reasoning will be, as we shall see, that 'virtue' means value, and is better off when thus expressed.)

The trouble with predication is that it can signify two radically different things. One is that a predicate (for example, justice or prudence or temperance) may be a situational judgment or characterization, quite particular in its application. This is the case when we say that John's marrying his mistress Judith was a just act, considering their circumstances and the foreseeable consequences. On the other hand, predication could be a claim that an act or an agent is by nature inherently possessed of some asserted quality which it contains as a *property*. This is the case when it is said that John's marrying his mistress is the just thing to do—i.e., that marrying one's mistress is, as such, just, whereas not marrying her is, as such, unjust—whatever the context and situation.

Predication in the first sense is grammatical, without prejudice as to whether what is predicated is intrinsic or extrinsic. The second sense is metaphysical (sc. ontological), assigning the quality to a class of actions rather than to an action in particular. The position I would take is that only the grammatical meaning of 'predicate' is viable and valid in the ethical analysis of moral acts. This kind of rigorous definition results when we remember that moralizing is, after all, a certain kind of philosophizing, i.e., philosophizing concerned with values and acts.

Perhaps the most primitive form of the notion of virtue as a property is to be found in the story of Jesus healing the woman with a hemorrhage, of how she was cured when she touched him. He noticed that "virtue" (a palpable power) had gone out of him. It could be used up, or at least temporarily lost. It was a phenomenon, empirically observable, experienceable. The power of it was there, whether or not it was perceived and understood. Lest we put all this down to a past primitive idea, to be found only in the pages of history or the reports of anthropologists, it is worth recalling that the same superstition survives in various forms in present-day cultures. Virtue for many people is objectively existent and is actually there, as *charisma* or *mana* is in some religious doctrines (for example, Catholic holy orders) and in some popular versions of political leadership, as noted by Max Weber ("He 'has' or 'possesses' a strong charisma.").[1]

Moral qualities or goodnesses or virtues are not properties, they are only predicates. That is, moral choices and acts do not contain, or subsist in, any necessary goodness or rightness. Moral quality is something that happens to be true of a human act; it is not given in the act itself but in the *gestalt* or situation. Right decisions and good deeds have to be so designated or nominated or judged—or, as Dewey preferred to say, appraised—to be such. Sometimes a lie is prudent, sometimes imprudent. Sometimes surrender to ruthless tyranny is cowardice, sometimes courage. Like martinis, marijuana may or may not be a bad thing. It all depends. No moral act is *bonum* or *malum in se*—only *per accidens, ex casu*. And this is because such terms as value and virtue and goodness and rightness denote what is not actual but conceptual, not real but nominal, not properly expressed as nouns but only as adjectives. It cannot be said that So-and-so or such-and-such "has" virtue. Moral quality is not reifiable. It is not a hypostatic entity.

The much too common idea, even among many philosophers, is that the goodness or value or virtue of things or acts is objectively real. For example, in a recent amusing book about the stock market, by a writer using the pseudonym "Adam Smith," the author says, "Value is there, like Bishop Berkeley's tree that made a noise when it fell in the forest whether or not anybody heard it fall. . ." The "old" objective morality held in effect that value or goodness is there whether anybody values it or not. It is my contention that physical or empirical facts are objective but values are subjective. A fallen tree sets up objectively knowable sound waves, whether aurally received or not; but whether it was good or bad would depend upon the receiver, not on the sound.

G. E. M. Anscombe, Wittgenstein's translator, is correct at least in her endorsement of his argument that the statements "this apple is red" and "this act is right" (good or virtuous) are not of the same order.[2] Moral propositions are evaluative, not descriptive. They are predicative, not substantive; they deal with nominal rather than "natural" entities. Russell's blunt claim, "In ethics there are no facts," is a scarecrow reduction of the question, but it is essentially correct. The "truth" of values or virtues has to be seen with the eyes of faith and known by approbation. Not by proof.

Moore embraced what he elected to call *intrinsic value,* but even so he acknowledged that to find any such value "it is necessary to consider what things are such that, if they existed by themselves, in absolute isolation, we should yet judge their existence to be good."[3] But this is an innocuous use of 'intrinsic' since nothing exists by itself in absolute isolation—not even God in any theistic metaphysics. Things are valuable or virtuous only because they are valued by a valuer, just as there must be a knower if a thing is to be known. Virtue is assigned by people, it is not resident in acts or things. What Dewey called the "transactional" theory of knowledge (the knower's always being involved or coinherent in the known) applies here too. Value (virtue) is transactional. It was Plato who started talk about "good itself" (*auto to agathon*) and it is high time we dropped it.

The "naturalistic fallacy" is the supposition that out of empirical data we can derive knowledge of what virtue is and what we ought to do. The heart of the matter, already to have been found in Hume's Razor (Max Black once called it a "guillotine"), is far more effectively and directly expressed by Karl Popper in his conclusion that nature "is in itself neither moral or immoral," and, "To sum up, *it is impossible to derive a sentence stating a norm or a decision or, say, a proposal for a policy from a sentence stating a fact.*"[4] Later, Hare put it even more succinctly: "No imperative conclusion can be validly drawn from a set of premises which does not contain at least one imperative."[5] "A moral judgment is then a decisional act, just in the sense that it is conceived as a determination which an individual human being makes for himself and as one for which there is no counterpart *in re.*"⁶ In the tersest statement of all, Sartre's, "We cannot possibly derive imperatives from ontology's indicatives."⁷

We can get the whole matter into the sharpest focus by turning from philosophers to sociologists. George Lundberg has said,

> It would be difficult to find a better example of confused thinking than that offered by the current discussion of 'values'... A principle cause of the confusion is a semantic error...It consists in converting the verb 'valuating,' meaning any discriminatory or selective behavior, into a noun called 'values.' We then go hunting for the things denoted by the noun. But there are no such things.⁸

We can use 'virtue' and 'value' interchangeably without altering what is being said. It really does not mean anything to say that good is better than evil, or that we ought to tell the truth, until and unless we convert such propositions into their operational or situational terms. Then, and only then, can we decide whether truth-telling is "good" and whether we "ought" to do it or not.

Given the view thus far developed of moral acts, what do they *do*? This question of their usefulness, which is decisive for their truth or goodness in both pragmatism and utilitarianism, arises with special interest or concern for all those who find the moral quality of deeds and conduct in the doing rather than in any classifying or categorizing of the deeds themselves. What virtuous acts do or effect is of pressing importance once we reject the notion that virtue is its own reward and accept the extrinsic view that virtues are contingent, not given. This is a consequential, or what Hare has called "supervenient," mode of moral judgment.

We all know the typological opposition: duties versus goals; ethics based on obedience to moral laws as opposed to ethics based on aspiration after an ideal or the desire to (as Moore put it) "optimize" some value or virtue, some standard or criterion of goodness. In actual practice, philosophers have tried to keep a foot in both boats—as is the case among some utilitarians, early and late, who try to argue that to obey a "summary rule" is to optimize general utility, or the greatest good of the greatest number. Even Moore said we ought to follow a general norm even though in a particular case it would be wrong (i.e., not useful), since left to ourselves we might judge the consequences erroneously. But this resorts to the rather threadbare ploys that (a) an occasional departure from a rule, for the sake of immediately good consequences, could be the "entering wedge" which will undermine the rule in its remote consequences, by encouraging indifference to the principle of the greatest good, and (b) such departures are "dangerous precedents" because people fear both in themselves and others a kind of savagery—"original sin"?—which will be strengthened by even the most constructive variances from the rule. The opinion that an action which is not customary or conventional is wrong or, if it is right, is a dangerous freedom, results in what Paul Freund has expressed as "the conclusion that nothing should be done for the first time!"[9]

There is a difference between a moral method based upon obedience to rules and one based upon the constant effort to realize values. The difference is what all the storied dilemmas illustrate: for example, whether to lie to the madman who is trying to find and kill an innocent person who he thinks is "hexing" him; or the captive who must violate a rule against suicide to keep vital information from falling into the hands of the enemy; or deciding for or against terminating a pregnancy to prevent a probable monstrosity. In cases such as these one cannot follow both a law-ethics and a goal-ethics.

In actuality the "rule utilitarians" (Toulmin, Baier, Nowell-Smith, et al.) are only arguing that it is improper linguistically to call a violation of a rule *right* or *just*. This, however, is a semantic objection in the psychological, not the logical sense—in a verbal rather than an analytical sense. Rightness or justice is not a matter of mere words, and their falling back on such a defense is a measure of the "restricted" utilitarians' uncomfortable position.[10] An ethically sound rule is, of course, framed on general utility or what is commonly conducive to "good" consequences for human needs and welfare. But it is contradictory to maintain a rule based on human benefit and at the same time to prohibit an act which is aimed at human benefit, unless it can be shown that there is a conflict between the good of the beneficiaries of the particular act and the legitimate interests of other human beings.

It is noteworthy that G. E. Moore of Cambridge based his acceptance of rules on an altogether different and less defensible ground. He feared that being rule-free might lead decision makers to error. (We can be sure that if they are human and finite, they will make mistakes sometimes.) But asking us to make moral decisions according to prefabricated rules— regardless of the relativities and realities of a concrete situation, simply because we might incorrectly judge the situation and mistakenly foretell the consequences of departing from the apparently relevant rule—is a doctrine of irrationality and intellectual irresponsibility utterly unworthy of Moore.

All of this means that we cannot make categorical virtues—of such contingent and derivative values as truth telling, promise keeping, life protecting, marriage preserving, virginity saving, nation defending, and the like. Our commitment to these rules must be hypothetical only. We will, for example, tell the truth when and if it serves or contributes to some good, some value, over and above and superior to the mere act— only if it furthers happiness, public safety, and the like. But these values are themselves, in their turn in the hierarchy of means and ends in one's value structure, subordinate or contributory to some *summum bonum*, to some highest good which is always to be served. It is this fixed ultimate standard which prevents ethical relativity from becoming ethical anarchy or chaos. This *summum bonum* is the only universal or "absolute" moral obligation, and any or all goods or values or virtues are or are not to be "acted out" or "done" only if and when the concrete situation causes them to serve the overall good or value or virtue—the singular general. In short, everything depends upon the consequences.

This "singular general" or formal principle or highest good can be labelled as 'general utility' or 'happiness' or 'the good of persons' or 'agapism' or 'human welfare'. What all of these terms contain in common is the belief that it is good to help people. Even agapism with its theological connotations holds that the only way to love God is through loving concern for people. The first-order value is the same. Utilitarians do not all define 'general utility' in the same operative terms; eudaemonists do not always agree about what happiness calls for; personists judge situations differently; agapists, no matter how much they share general rules, often find different acts required for love's sake in specific cases. Even simple humanism (Dewey's, for example) does not guarantee that its exponents will make the same "instrumental" decisions in a given situation. Moral rules are to be used heuristically, to illuminate and suggest, not with apodictic literalism to prescribe a course out of obedience to a formal rule of conduct.

For these reasons what virtues do is to provide guidelines, illuminating maxims. They generalize experience for the serious and careful decision maker. What they do not do is decide the act by abstract prescription; they are not rules or laws to be obeyed. They are tentative bearings which the responsible moral agent takes into account as he chooses the course of action offering the consequences most favorable to his highest good or virtue, generically understood—call it utility or happiness or love or *blik*.

We are now in a position to say intelligibly that virtue (as distinguished from and paramount to "the virtues") should displace duty in the choice of moral acts. This is the same as saying, in the formal language of ethics, that we should be teleological or concerned with consequences, not deontological or obedient to rules and laws. The goal of moral action is not to obey any Euclidian theorems deduced from it as general rules. Or, obversely, we ought to obey or follow the logic of virtue in the singular general without being straitjacketed by any specific virtues in the plural particular. If anybody needs the word *duty* let him attach it to moral goal seeking if he wants and feels better doing so. If he likes the *word*, let him ignore the analytic objections outlined and call teleology his duty. At least he is free of rules as moral prisons.

Kant poured out his scorn on the ethics of hedonism and ended up with a howling instance of legalism. He held that no conception of virtue (for example, of loving concern or human happiness or personal fulfillment or social justice) would be any better than the value judgment that physical pleasure is the highest good. In short, his conclusion was that virtue is the same thing as obeying moral laws or rules. Thus he reflected the deontological moralism of the Jewish-Christian-Stoic tradition. And because for Kant obedience was categorically imperative, what he was really saying in a circular way was that we should obey rules because we should. This will not stand up under either empirical or analytical scrutiny. Kant, like all legalists (deontologists), was saying that if you love your neighbor you are not virtuous, but if you tell him the truth even though you despise him you are virtuous.[11]

Starting at least as early as Samuel Clarke and John Balguy and coming up to A. C. Ewing in our own times, there have been a few ethicists who have sought to slip out from between the deontic and telic positions. Their conception of the moral act is a fitting response to a situation. Clarke and Balguy were explicitly agapistic about it; the fitting response is the one that acts out or effects a loving concern in the intended consequences. Ewing is far less explicit, much more implicitly agapistic—preferring a number of value terms more or less equivalent to love.[12]

What is meant by a fitting or appropriate act is, of course, whatever in the concrete situation seems most consistent with the ideal or criterion or standard held by the moral agent—be it sheer self-advantage, social concern (agape), a romantic or interpersonal loyalty, national interest, whatever value is the highest good and ruling first-order consideration. This kind of ethical method is not committed to doing what is right in the conventional sense of obeying a rule. Rather, it aims at acting in such a way as to do the good (i.e., acting with the situational logic of its *summum bonum*) regardless of rules and goals.

In fact, this "third force" method is, after all, only a version of teleology. Certainly it is not duty- or rule-centered. But neither is it goal-centered in the sense of being unwaveringly devoted to a proximate goal (like national power or personal ambition). It is, however, teleological in the proper and basic sense; that is, it aims situationally at optimizing a highest good which is less proximate, more ultimate and ulterior— e.g., happiness or human welfare.

To act creatively or constructively, i.e., morally, it is necessary to choose to act according to goals rather than rules. Rule ethics are duty ethics, law ethics, deontology. Act or situation ethics are goal ethics, ideal or virtue ethics, teleology. My aim is to interpret goodness teleologically, as we have seen—in terms of faithfulness to values instead of to rules. And ultimately this means faithfulness to a first-order value, a highest good, rather than to any specific or derivative values (or virtues).

As a eudaemonist to whom happiness meant self-realization, Aristotle's ideal was the Good Man. (Incidentally, this was not the Good Fellow of the cook-out crowd in suburbia or their downtown rendezvous at the Rotary luncheon. Popular or customary morality is by definition mimetic and, therefore, leans toward rules or codes.) It is largely due to Aristotle's great influence in Western ethics, both theological and non-theological, that so much attention has focused upon character. Many moralists have laid their emphasis on the crucial role of the agent, rather than upon moral rules or upon the agent's judgments in specific acts or particular situations. After all, virility and virtue both come from *vir*, 'man'.

This tradition reminds us that we can speak in a meaningful way, not simply of rules versus decision as the rival keys to moral acts, but of disposition as well. It is certainly true that in some highly problematic situations in which the rules are either not apparent or are in conflict (what classical casuistry called 'doubt' and 'perplexity'), or where the decision maker operates with an ethical model based on values rather than rules and yet cannot clearly see his course, what then is really decisive or crucial—what counts—is the agent's character or predisposition. In such a case what is practically important is the good man, not the good rule or the good judgment.[13]

But we all know that the road to hell is paved with good intentions. This old adage calls attention to the regrettable fact that good character does not automatically produce good acts. Being well disposed has a necessary or at least predispositional relation to the agent's values, but not to a right act—right, that is, in accordance with his values. Reliance upon character to lead to right acts is no doubt related to such sayings as Jiminy Cricket's in *Pinocchio*, "Let your conscience be your guide." This is the notion that conscience is not reason making moral judgments (as Thomas Aquinas said) but a kind of built-in moral radar (as in guidance-doctrines or, on the other hand, in intuition theory), or as something not built-in but built-up—i.e., acquired or developed. The overlap between conscience—in these conventional senses—and character is obvious.

In classical moral theology it has been held that virtues are dispositions of the will, by which it was meant that they are values or desirables which the agent is willing to serve or seek or optimize. In the Catholic ethos, it would be fair to say, the stress has been on teleology or aspiration, i.e., on the attainment of virtuous character—with the not altogether naive expectation that it will result in good deeds. This compares, of course, with the Protestant ethos in which the stress has been deontological, i.e., on obedience to rules. Perhaps we need not go any deeper in explaining the difference than just to point to Protestantism's greater emphasis on "sin" and even on a "fallenness" understood as *tota depravatio.*

However, just as the theologians emphasized generic sin ("original sin") rather than specific sins in their attempts to account for vicious, as opposed to virtuous, dispositions of the will, we would be well advised to stress virtuous dispositions of the will rather than specific "virtues." Let specific virtues be what a loving or humane disposition of the will selects in concrete and particular situations. Virtue, then, is a good disposition of the will, a teleological force, and acts are decisions of the will thus disposed.

The moral agent's big danger, teleologically speaking, is that he will be chained by traditions and rules, making the virtue of no effect. The new breed of young people who speak of a "new morality" have as their maxim, "Hang loose, Baby." They are on the right track. (It may be well argued, of course, that they do not sufficiently appreciate the wisdom of some moral rules, but whether they do or not they ought not to be bound invariably or unexceptionably by any of them.) And this is because basically no act is inherently good or virtuous or "right" merely because of its kind. It is only virtuous if it optimizes the agent's virtue in the particular situation—i.e., if it facilitates the most or greatest good possible then and there, measured or calculated in terms of foreseeable consequences both immediate and remote. Concise generalizations (Lying undermines human relations) are acceptable, but precise specifications (Never lie to a dying patient) are unacceptable.

What is of determinative importance, as befits an ethics on the teleological model, is consequences. Here we can stand shoulder to shoulder with Moore and all other utilitarians and pragmatists. What justifies an act is its results, not its conformity to moral rules. The logic of consequentialism is, of course, that the end justifies the means.[14] (Moore, remember, called the denial of this "utterly false," and so it is.) Doing evil in order that a preponderant good may come means doing what is by rule wrong (even sometimes a wise rule) because the good or desired potential consequences in the situation outweigh the evil; it is a question of what the casuists have always called 'proportionate good'. Kant said that to will the end is to will the means, and we may paraphrase him: To will the consequences is to will the means. Jewish and Christian moralists have held that we may never do evil for good's sake, that we should prefer evil consequences to violating a moral rule. In so holding, however, they are really saying that freedom and the responsible calculation of benefits is to be left to God alone. All theological solutions of the problem of evil in a divinely ordered world are based on the claim that out of evil God brings good.

It seems plain, given our extrinsic or "approbative" view of goodness, that values are a better model for moral decision making than rules. Coupled with consideration of consequences as the merit-test, the result is situation ethics or a contextual relativism. Let me offer, then, a brief account of what it means, in these terms, to do right or to choose the right act.

Brand Blanshard tells of a conversation with Moore in which the latter said, "It still seems to me self-evident that we always ought so to act as to produce the greatest good, that is, to make the world as much better as we can." This reflects William James, almost to the words.[15] Blanshard adds, "This is the supreme maxim of the teleologists, the categorical imperative that they believe holds without exception: So to act as to produce the greatest good. Here I follow them." He says further, "On the actual consequences of our acts their objective rightness depends. On their intended consequences depends their subjective rightness."[16]

The point is that goodness is moral quality or worth, while rightness is a moral act-judgment. Consequences can be good in the sense that they are worthy, and the agent can be good in the sense that he aims at such consequences of his actions, but the actions are either right or wrong (correct or faulty) according to his success or failure to effect the intended consequences. We can put it as Moore did, "that 'right' does and can mean nothing but 'cause of a good result' and is thus identical with 'useful'."[17]

The situational relativity of moral decisions may be expressed as a syllogism. In decision making the major premise expresses the situation or reality context, and the minor premise asserts a value proposition. Logical reasoning and empirical realism provide the conclusion. The minor premise or value proposition is valid only relative to the situation—it is not absolutely or objectively or constantly valid (i.e., obliging).

In a game of bridge a good general rule is that the third hand plays high, but if my partner leads with the ace should I play my king? Possibly, though not probably; "right" is contingent, not constant or inherent in any ethical game. Just as the virtuous or loving or good thing to aim at will vary according to situations, so the right act must therefore vary too. Only the ideal or *summum bonum* is constant; situations are variables, and they make operational values or sought consequences variables too. This is what moral theologians have called a "prudential application of principle."

This relativity of moral acts makes facts or data vitally important. We have to reject the "naturalistic fallacy"—any suggestion that facts can yield values (*is* won't produce *ought*). Nevertheless, ethical naturalism has this much validity, that the data determines or shapes which *oughts* and, teleologically, how much and when and where *oughts* should be aimed. We need, as Dewey said, not only to "prize" consequences but to "appraise" situations. Situationists more than any others take seriously the maxim, Nobody's opinions are any better than his facts. To see the core truth that sometimes a lie is right and sometimes a lie is wrong, and to assign this relativity to any and all rules of conduct or normative principles, denying them their allegedly prescriptive and apodictic force, is reason indeed to be as well informed as possible, to take situations with the utmost seriousness. As somebody (I think it was James) once said, monists are apt to say "all," but pluralists say "each."

Konrad Lorenz, the Austrian ethologist, speaks of "injunctive definition," meaning definition in terms of many constituent characteristics and factors—none of which by itself constitutes the thing defined, but which taken together do. This applies to a situationist's approach to moral situations. It suggests that we need more description, less definition. Injunctive definition is, indeed, description. Definition falsifies because it tends to fix things and to treat ingredients and components as given, as properties. And this, as we said to begin with, is the root or cardinal ethical error. Its source is probably psychological, a distate for or actual fear of the task of constant decision, and a hunger for authority and pretailored decisions (rules). Too often the moral choice is not easy or obvious, and the *ratio decidendi* seems too perilous. It is this burden of moral decision and moral autonomy which Sartre calls the source of man's *angoisse*, his existential anxiety.

The ancients like Aristotle and Augustine discussed ethics in terms of virtue and virtues, i.e., values, and only later in the Middle Ages and Reformation did rules become the foci of analysis. Even in classical Christian moral theology some "systems" are based on the cardinal virtues (temperance, fortitude, prudence, and justice) and the theological virtues (faith, hope and love), while more recently developed systems—the Jesuits', for example—are based on rules, the Decalogue. Once we abandon the rules-model we find ourselves again with the values-model.

Thomas Aquinas puts it all succinctly:

> Disquisitions on general morality are not entirely trustworthy, and the ground becomes more uncertain when one wishes to descend to individual cases in detail. The factors are infinitely variable, and cannot be settled either by art or precedent. Judgment should be left to the people concerned. Each must set himself to act according to the immediate situation and the circumstances involved. The decision may be unerring in the concrete, despite the uneasy debate in the abstract. Nevertheless, the moralist can provide some help and direction in such cases.[18]

Reviewing his own pursuit of reason in ethics, Stephen Toulmin found that it was a finite chain of "because" and "it follows" and "therefores". "In any case," he said, "a point was reached beyond which it was no longer possible to give 'reasons' of the kind given until then; and eventually there came a stage beyond which it seemed no 'reason' of any kind could be given." He is, of course, speaking of value-choices—i.e., metaethical or metamoral data, chosen rather than being logically necessary. They are, we might say, legitimate and necessary instances of logical vacuity. Such, indeed, are all first-order values or ideals. Toulmin calls them "limiting" and quotes Wittgenstein's remark about such questions: "This is a terrible business—just terrible. You can at best stammer when you talk of it."[19] This stammering is the business of faith and decision, not of facts and conclusions. It is, as in theology, the foundation of ethics—whether the ethics be cognitive or noncognitive, objective or approbative. All systems or methods start with value, and value is a personal affirmation, not a fact-conclusion.

Gilbert Ryle once pointed out that if we are to resolve or find an "armistice" in the war between religion and science, it will have to be "not from making compromises but only from drawing uncompromising contrasts between their businesses."[20] The same applies to ethical judgments and empirical statements. Theologizers, with their faith, should be prepared to jettison whatever science can falsify, and the same should apply to moralizers. But neither faith nor morals can get their substance from data; they can only use data to regulate their use of their beliefs and their values.

In the end, the business of ethics always comes back to persons, to decision makers. Each one of us has to decide (a) what to do, and (b) why. Even if a person, a responsible individual, tries to live and act by precooked beliefs and moral acts (as provided by church, state, party, gang, or any other "authority") he still has to decide whether he will accept them. Precooked morality is a false morality and a philosophical cuckoo's nest, but in spite of its attraction for the weary or the weak it still forces its adherents to decide for or against it. We have to decide, even if it is a decision not to decide. Nondecision (law ethics) is sub-human.

1. Work by Frazer, Goldenweiser and Kelsen has described *mana*. Various authors in a symposium by Cambridge divines [*Traditional Virtues Reassessed*, ed. Alec R. Vilder, (London: S.P.C.K., 1964)] speak of virtue as a thing "given." Being pious, they say it is a "possession," a "gift" of grace, something to be "acquired." Christian theologians reify "grace" too, speaking of it as a substance which is "poured out" and "carried" or "transmitted."

2. Expressed *viva voce* at an ethics workshop at the Catholic University of America, Washington, June, 1968.

3. G. E. Moore, *Principia Ethica* (Cambridge: Cambridge University Press, 1960), 187.

4. Karl R. Popper, *The Open Society and Its Enemies* (Princeton, N.J.: Princeton University Press, 1950), 65. Popper's italics.

5. R. M. Hare, *The Language of Morals* (Oxford: Oxford University Press, 1952), 28.

6. F. A. Olafson, *The Ethical Interpretation of Existentialism* (Baltimore: Johns Hopkins University Press, 1967), 140-141.

7. Jean-Paul Sartre, *Being and Nothingness* (New York: Philosophical Library, 1956), 625.

8. George Lundberg, *Can Science Save Us?*, 2nd ed. (New York: Longmans, Green and Company, 1961), 30.

9. Paul Freund, *On Law and Justice* (Cambridge: Harvard University Press, 1968), 155, quoting F. M. Cornford's *Microcosmographia Academica* (Chicago: University of Chicago Press, 1945).

10. See M. G. Singer, *Generalization in Ethics* (New York: Alfred A. Knopf, Inc., 1961), *passim*. Historians still disagree as to whether Mill was, like Bentham, a rule utilitarian.

11. What an odd inconsistency that Kant, given his contempt for pleasure, should have argued for God's existence on the ground that it would be unjust if the good should suffer in the end; an ultimate reward must be eternal life guaranteed pleasant by an unmockable God. This "moral" argument was popular in the nineteenth century.

12. A. C. Ewing, *The Definition of the Good* (New York: The Macmillan Company, 1947). A contemporary nontheological ethicist who is explicitly agapistic is G. C. Field, *Moral Theory* (London: Methuen and Company, 1966).

13. Agent ethics, distinguished from act ethics, would subordinate decision making to character building, and minimize the calculations of consequences.

14. Said John Dewey, "Certainly nothing can justify or condemn means except ends, results." "Yet," he adds, we ought also "to note the plural effects that flow from any act": "Not *the* end—in the singular—justifies the means; for there is no such thing as the single all-important end." *Human Nature and Conduct* (New York: Henry Holt and Company, 1922) 147, 228-229. Dewey is saying that *proportionate* good must decide, in view of the "package" of immediate, remote, and concomitant consequences.

15. William James, *The Moral Philosopher and the Moral Life*. James said, "There is but one unconditional commandment, which is that we should seek incessantly, with fear and trembling, so to vote and so to act as to bring about the very largest total universe of good which we can see."

16. Brand Blanshard, *Ethics and Society*, ed. R. T. DeGeorge (New York: Doubleday and Company, 1966), 10-11.

17. G. E. Moore, *Principia Ethica* (Cambridge: Cambridge University Press, 1960), 147.

18. Thomas Aquinas, *Commentary on Aristotle's Ethics*, Bk. II, Lect. 2 (brought to my attention by Albert DiAnni, SM, Marist College and Seminary, Framingham Centre, Massachusetts).

19. Stephen Toulmin, *Reason and Ethics* (Cambridge: Cambridge University Press, 1960), 32.

20. Gilbert Ryle, *Dilemmas* (Cambridge: Cambridge University Press, 1954), 81.

Four

Distributive Justice

As we have seen, values are the necessary parameters of moral judgments. Literally speaking, they are the quality standards or measures we set alongside a moral act to judge its rightness or wrongness. In mathematical language, they are the independent variables we use in any set of ethical equations.

At first this may sound too strangely mathematical to be appropriate to ethical discourse, not fitting for the study of the moral qualities of good and evil. I confess that my own training in philosophical and theological ethics was deeply planted in the humanities, with the consequence that I, like many others of my breed, feel uncomfortable and incompetent whenever questions of distribution and the requisite quantifiers are raised. All the same, the main purpose of this chapter is to contend that any serious ethical analysis of health care delivery plunges us headlong and unavoidably into what I can only call ethical arithmetic.

The mere phrase "ethical arithmetic" revives memories of the way seventeenth-century economists like Petty and North spoke of "political arithmetic." Any social inquiry, ethics included, has to calculate quantities.

Controversy or disputation can be either good or bad, depending on whether its payoff comes down to more light or more heat. T. P. O'Connor once said, "If only the Catholics and Protestants in Ireland were all good pagans we could get along like Christians." In some controversies there is too much heat, too little light. However, even though we hope that light and understanding will follow from the abrasions of ethical discourse, it is still true that the best model for ethical discourse is incandescent light. Incandescence, from sunlight to the filament in an electric light bulb, comes from heat. The heat always needs minimizing and controlling, but it can never be entirely dispensed with.

Ethics is as much concerned with social questions as with personal questions. One such issue about which men have always argued is distributive justice, or the right way to allocate limited or scarce resources. Finite resources are a worrisome problem in all areas, but nowhere more so than in medicine and health care. Even with the greatest potential of "socialized medicine" theoretically, there are limits on what can be provided. Suppose we look at the problems of health policy as an example of distributive justice.

Economists and physicians warn us that "health dollars" are limited. We shall always have to decide who should be treated and who should not, who shall die and who shall live. Can we as a society afford, for example, the recent Federal artificial kidney treatment that costs $60,000 *a year* for each patient—at present a billion dollars for 50,000 people? What about other unmet needs? What about the values of *preventive* medicine? What is a just cut-off point in providing health care?

The best definition of health is the World Health Organization's. It is far more analytic and comprehensive than the individualistic and one-to-one definition with which clinical medicine has functioned historically. WHO defines health as *a complex of physical, mental, and social well-being*: all three. Yet Dr. John Knowles of the Rockefeller Foundation has charged, "The medical ostrich has buried its head in the sands of biological science and turned its backside to the major social issues of medical care today."[1]

In ethical language this means, it seems to me, that medical centers ought to be converted into health centers. Truly to understand the biomedical enterprise in terms of human well-being instead of in terms of physical health is a fairly radical proposal, even in the 1970s, because it broadens and deepens the obligations (a key ethical term) of health care to include treatment not only of mental disorders but of social causation too.

WHO's definition was anticipated a long time ago in the bureaucratic rhetoric of medical reports and public health literature. But even so, the only branch of medicine to date actually to take mental and social well-being into account, as well as physicial health, is cosmetic surgery!

In fact, physicians have tried steadily and stubbornly to keep the practice of medicine loose from psychology and psychiatry, and from public health management. Psychiatry or psychiatric medicine is still only a cousin in conventional medical sentiments, and certainly not a "kissin' cousin" yet. From the medical citadel public health workers are looked at as only very distant relatives, not in the cousin class at all. Sociologists are as scarce as ethicists in medical schools.

In any realistic view there is a nearly complete divorce of scientific and clinical medicine from the social and economic disciplines. This is the case educationally, institutionally, and ideologically. For example, schools of public health were separated a long time ago from medical education.

Biomedical thinking, it seems, is in greater flux right now than ever before, and this may mean that the well-being concept of medicine has a good chance of prevailing. This flux or creative disorder in medical rethinking is due to three major factors in health care change: (1) the expansion (not to say explosion) of medical knowledge through science; (2) the institution of social welfare programs, including various forms of prepaid medical care; and (3) the development of our present forms of medical education.

Looking back at the Greek experience, we find three models of health care. One was the Cult of the Dogmatists (i.e., the medical teachings of Pythagoras and Empedocles) based on metaphysical rather than pragmatic principles. This was what Hippocrates broke away from, in favor of etiology and natural causation and in revolt against the priests and Neoplatonists. The second was what they called the Cult of Aesculapius, a strictly one-to-one, patient-physician affair aimed at getting the particular individual physically well. The Aesculapian is still the real model of medicine ideologically, not only in the AMA but in medical schools also. The third one was what the Greeks called the Cult of Hygeia, the cult of the daughter of Aesculapius, which was a social or public health model of prevention as well as therapy.

Hygiene means "good for health." In the hygienic model prevention, rather than treatment, of disease is the *summum bonum*, and the problem of human well-being is understood and approached socially rather than privately or individually.

This hygienic model of the biomedical disciplines and of health care is presupposed in this chapter. It is the public health or public interest way of looking at the ethics of health care and its delivery to patients—patients who are seen not as paying customers privately contracted, but as consumers with a common concern and a collective need.

Even at the clinical level there are many ways in which delivery of health care in modern times poses new moral questions. For example, have husbands a valid moral claim ("right") to be present at the birth of their babies? The Montana Supreme Court, for one, ruled that they do not. Yet Dad's presence at delivery, as in the Lamaze or psychoprophylactic method of childbirth, is held by many to be essential to providing good obstetrical health care. Again, there are any number of ethical questions raised about various items in the Patient's Bill of Rights lately promulgated by the American Hospital Association. Such issues are all a part of the "consumerist" perspective on medicine, being spelled out more or less militantly in terms of consumer protection and patients' rights.

Hormone therapy, especially for minors, raises questions of right and wrong when, as is frequently a consequence of the treatment, the patient experiences an increase of sexual vigor almost compulsive in its force. And speaking of minors, what of the delivery of health care in the form of birth control (contraception, sterilization, and abortion) to minors, bypassing parental consent, which is now the practice under "mature minor" statutes in some states? As one example of the morality of health care delivery at the *clinical* level, how are we to formulate the ethics of surrogate therapy—the provision of psychiatrically supervised sex practice with therapeutic partners for patients with impotence, frigidity, inexperience, phobias, and so forth?

Such clinical problems of judgment and decision making, arresting as they are on their own level, are not the focus of this discussion. The social issues of health care delivery take shape more pointedly at the systems or programmatic level. Being neither a medical sociologist nor a public administrator, I lack the competence to do much more than indicate them, yet it is here that the essentially *social* nature of health care becomes manifest, and it is this *social* character or dimension that lies at the heart of this chapter.

It is precisely here, in the social dimension of medicine, that we run into the question of distributive justice, and distributive justice is the core or key question for biomedical ethics. Distributive justice is the biggest or most all-embracing ethical problem. Ultimately, the reputation of biomedical ethics is at stake in whether it deals with it or not, and in how it deals with it.

Since Aristotle we have distinguished between three orders of justice: commutative, legal, and distributive. It is still a meaningful typology. Commutative justice deals with what is due between persons, as in professional ethics, trade or market morality, the ethics of sex, family, and human reproduction—all problems of obligation in one-to-one and group relations. Legal justice has to do with what we as individuals owe to the community and to the state, in terms of jurisprudence, civil and criminal law, taxation, and the like. Distributive justice is concerned with what society and the state owe to individuals, as in public services and public utilities, protection of the environment, and—our special concern here—health care.

At this point, I enter an area in which I not only have had no training or experience, but where I find myself drawn to a conclusion that makes me decidedly uncomfortable. My conditioning in the grand tradition has instilled in me a "feeling" that values are one thing and numbers (digits or dollars) are something else. All ethics, however, should be based as the scientific ethic is, on honesty, and therefore like Martin Luther, I'll go where my understanding takes me. "I can do no other." Like Wittgenstein on values, I approach the *allocation* of values with Kierkegaard's "fear and trembling."

It seems that the heart of the problem of distributive justice is how we are to allocate our resources; for example, as between rural and urban patients; or between preventive and curative care; or between care by physicians and care by auxiliary and paramedical personnel; or between high-cost specialties and low-cost care. What the Chinese have done under the banner of "barefoot medicine," using lay trainees, is a specter haunting the old guard who want to hold the line for arcane medicine. Health maintenance organizations have run into massive resistance by the medical establishment. But given a serious commitment to exploring these options, what reallocations of roles and funds would distributive justice require?

Two of the most fiercely fought issues in the United States lately have had to do with health insurance proposals and peer review or monitoring of the quality of medical practice. PSROs (Professional Standards Review Organizations) were a matter of civil law by 1972, but bitterly opposed for two more years nonetheless, by doctors who did not want their performances checked out. (The House of Delegates of the AMA meeting June 26, 1974, in Chicago finally voted, 185 to 57, to support the PSRO law.) Yet it is obvious that monitoring is needed. One doctor in Massachusetts was found to be doing eighty disc operations per year—as many as are done at Massachusetts General Hospital by all the surgeons combined.

The screams of outrage against PSROs from the AMA have an ironic sound, since the AMA got its start as a peer review organization 125 years ago, to expose diploma mills, quacks, and financial highbinders. Peer review is, of course, what goes on anyway in any teaching hospital or university medical center.

Almost certainly the preponderant ethical issue about the delivery of medical care lies in rival proposals for national health insurance. The salient fact in all of this is the public's anger at the ruinous cost of medical care. Medicine is in trouble and its self-image in immediate jeopardy because it has been priced out of the marketplace. From 1960 to 1974 the cost of living rose by 52.2 percent while physicians' fees rose 57.7 percent and daily hospital charges went up from $56 to $144—up 155 percent.

Now that the picture has been painted what about it? Not being an economist, a statistician, or a political scientist, I cannot speak to the question which of these plans and options and distributions is most fair, most just. Justice cannot work without numbers; that much is obvious. It seems to me that the task of both the just man and of the legislature is, precisely, to choose whatever course would realize the greatest good of the greatest number—in this case, in the matter of health care.

Yet the question still remains, how is this ethical imperative to be put into effect? How are we to get the correct number, the hard data, in making value choices? It is on this point that I want to put my emphasis. Let me start by remarking that many of our historical modes of ethical thought are utterly *out*moded.

The scope and arena of ethical choice or preference have widened enormously since the days when being one's brother's keeper and loving one's neighbor was a direct matter between you and a handful of people personally known to you, in what anthropologists call a "primary community." The pastoral-agrarian and village society of the Bible no longer exists in our Atlantic civilization. We cannot continue to turn simplistically to the teachings of Moses or Jesus or Mohammed for direct ethical guidance. Things are just not that simple any more.

Ethics is perforce "social ethics" now. It is no longer, or at least less and less, what we might call interpersonal morality. The world is so tied together, due to the interdependence of technology and rapid transport, and to the density of urban culture steadily aggravated by irrational reproduction, that even the words "neighbor" and "stranger" are nearly archaic. We are caught in a tight web of radical interconnectivity.

What is needed is a moral telescope to see our moral problems through, not a moral microscope only. This is an age of macroethical more than microethical analysis. In medicine we have to deal with many patients who coexist, for instance, not just with patients one at a time. Hans Jonas says, "In the course of treatment the physician is obligated to the patient and no one else."[2] That, alas, is the classical ethic at its most myopic. It looks at the problem of medical care through a rear-view mirror.

The ancient one-to-one medical ethic is too simple, and it therefore falsifies ethical problems. A moral calculus of some kind is required if we are to cope justly with the imperative of health care delivery. Along with the one-to-one ethic we can set aside other classical norms as outmoded and therefore actually unethical—for example, such vestigial bits of medical piety as "first come, first served," "*non nocere*, do no harm," and the "inviolability of medical secrets."

Any very sophisticated discussion of social justice and the delivery of health care is rich with such terms as priorities, relative claims, triage, value judgment, systems analysis, allocation of scarce resources, cost-benefit balance, tradeoff, games theory, decision making, choice, options. This is what I take to be the contemporary and relevant language of ethics. As an ethical lexicon, it predicates quantifiers, numbers, and weights. Ethical judgments need, somehow, to quantify qualities or to measure values.

Daniel Callahan was on target quoting Kenneth Boulding's definition, "A moral, or ethical, proposition is a statement about a rank order of preferences among alternatives, which is intended to apply to more than one person."[3] Whether the weights we assign to different values and interests in our ethical mix are monetary or arithmetical, somehow we must learn to actually program computers with preference questions.

Robert Theobald, the Anglo-American economist, told a symposium at Vanderbilt University in 1971, "If you pulled the plug on the computers this country would come to a grinding halt." I have a feeling that Theobald is right. If so, this would mean that artificial intelligence is the only answer to the magnitude of human relations in a technological world of runaway material production and human reproduction.

We are all fairly familiar with trade-off and cost-benefit judgment at the clinical level, and the notion of proportionate good, in so-called triage decisions. Selection committees face it in renal programs where patients outnumber the perfusion slots available on kidney machines. This can be difficult, of course, as when, for example, the choice is between a candidate with good prospects versus a patient already in dialysis with a neurosurgical deficit, such as the loss of frontal lobes, or maybe one with hemorrhage of the GI tract.

But this gets a lot more *statistical* when we look at an uptown New York hospital's ethical question about its relative obligations. Its hyperbaric chamber cost $750,000 to install, $600,000 per year to operate. In five years the total cost was $3,700,000—and only 900 patients were treated, at a cost of $4111.11 each. For the same amount of money, twenty thousand outpatients could have been treated per year, or one hundred thousand altogether. Or a screening program could have been set up in East Harlem to detect lead poisoning and anemia in a million children, to keep their brains from being ruined. If you want to think about ethics and health care delivery, here is a good case, posing all the factors at stake—both numbers and competing values.

The numbers question gets lots harder when hundreds and thousands are involved, not just two or ten. There is the famous story about the medical corps problem in North Africa during the Second World War. Penicillin was in short supply. It could be used to treat a few hundred badly wounded soldiers, or it could be used in light dosages for several thousand who were out of action only because of venereal disease caught in brothels in the rest areas.

The American military's health care policy in front line stations is to give priority of treatment to those with minor health problems rather than overwhelmingly serious wounds. The United States government's civil defense policy in the event of nuclear war is the same—lightly injured first, badly injured last.

This is utilitarian ethics—the greatest good of the greatest number. But it would be a pity if our discussion got bogged down in a doctrinaire debate over the theoretical strengths and weaknesses of utilitarianism. As a question on its own merits it would be an important subject, but in the present context I believe the main thing is the problem of distributive justice and when we should or should not maximize the recipients of health care or optimize the quality of the health care delivered. The utilitarians are in the picture inevitably, since from the start they set their sights and based their ethics on the public welfare and justice, as in Jeremy Bentham's *Principles of Morals and Legislation*; they "politicized" ethics. But we can avoid a lot of energy loss by simply heeding Albert Jonsen's advice: "Ethics must learn to speak the language of public policy in order to function as easily in conference rooms and legislative halls as in the classroom."[4]

In Britain it was argued that contraceptive pills would cause embolisms because of the estrogen—which was true. But the health service persisted for the reason that fourteen such deaths per million users is preferable to 228 deaths per million nonusers—deaths, that is, resulting from pregnancy and childbirth. Since the mortality rate is seventeen times higher for pregnancies than for contraception, it acted for the greater good of the greater number.

This kind of mathematics only gathers and compares numbers, however. When we have to compare values as well as sums, which is the real problem of ethical arithmetic or mathematical morality, then things begin to get hazier and harder. Look, for example, at a problem of health care delivery faced by WHO and the government of Sri Lanka. The anopheles mosquito spreads fast in Ceylon, but by DDT spraying they cut malaria cases from 2.8 million in 1961 to only 110 cases in 1964 (three years' time). Appreciating that DDT does ecological damage, they then stopped spraying, in the belief that the pests were licked. The mosquitos returned at once; in 1968-69 malaria had again infected 2.5 million people.

Here is an ethical choice problem comprising both numbers and values. The numbers are easy, but how should we relate the values of ecologic balance to human mortality rates? It is my belief that this task of value ranking must itself be converted into numbers, dollars, or abstract digits, or whatever, before we will be able to quantify the moral options we have to program into our computers' data banks. Without it we cannot optimize the widest benefit (the nonmoral good) at stake in health care delivery, nor make the most favorable calculations needed if the ideal we serve is human well-being for all.

Here, then, is the heart of this chapter—that we must set out on a new task for ethics, an effort to innovate a mathematical morality or statistical ethics. Gordon Rattray Taylor put it neatly when he said we lack "a mathematics of mercy" with which to "calculate who, of thousands of sufferers, should receive the privilege of being saved by scarce facilities."[5] The ethics of delivery health care requires us to face the realities of a finite world, the fact that growth and resources have limits. John Stuart Mill made this perfectly clear 150 years ago in his essay on the stationary state, and more recently it was brought home by the Club of Rome, in the English *Ecologist's* "Blueprint for Survival," and by the Meadows's *Limits of Growth*.

In 1961, there was a brief debate between Warren Weaver of the Rockefeller Foundation and Roger Shinn of the Union Seminary:[6] Weaver pointed out that the "five principle world religions of revelation" got their start too long ago to have much to say about our interdependent modern world. Our problem now is cost-benefit judgments about things like new expressways or highrise building construction when weighed against the predictable loss of life entailed. Accurate projective estimates by so-called actuaries are available and reliable. Trade-off decisions of this kind go on all the time in medicine, transport, building, mining, everything.

Shinn argued, on the other hand, that "some aspects of ethics can never be reduced to statistics." As his example he took Jesus' nomadic-agrarian parable about the lost sheep and the shepherd who left ninety-nine sheep in the wilderness to hunt the one that was lost. Shinn's idea was that you cannot relativize the value of some things, such as a human life. But surely it would be unjust if leaving the flock actually risked losing ninety-nine for one. (Many exegetes say there was, in fact, no such risk.) He tried further to sharpen the issue by asking Ivan's question in Dostoevski's *Brothers Karamazov*: Would it be justifiable to make all men happy at the cost of torturing one little baby to death? If in this hypothetical case the world's unhappiness included the disease and deaths of countless people, then of course trading one for many would be hypothetically right—the preponderance of good over evil, of benefit over cost.

Is it morally justifiable to choose and make preferences not only between things but between people? Can we ethically decide that one patient is "worth" more than another or has a greater claim to medical care? You might think that the answer is obviously yes, but there are some who would challenge you. In my own living room one evening the question was posed in terms of the selection problem in organ transplants. However difficult, ought we to choose between patients of equal medical acceptability, if not all can be treated? A surgeon, an ethics teacher, a retired American Telephone and Telegraph executive, and I agreed that we should indeed choose, but the fifth member of the party, dean of a theological school, said no. "All human beings," he argued, "are infinitely precious in God's eyes, of equal worth and dignity, and therefore to be selective would be to play God."

He would not, he explained, choose between an Einstein's life and a low-grade moron's. It is clear that the dean was thinking absolutistically, in terms of a sanctity-of-life ethics. For him a life was intrinsically good, regardless of relativities, and therefore any one life was as valuable as any other.

A debate at the University of Virginia between a religion professor and a specialist in renal medicine highlighted this issue. Professor James Childress argued that no nonmedical or personal criteria should be considered; in cases where some are chosen rather than others, the decision should be based on chance or lottery. Dr. Frederick Westervelt argued that selection procedures would be "derelict" if they did not as rationally as possible seek the "most suitable" of the medically suitable.

Besides these two notions of how to cope with choice problems—by resort to chance and by analytic selection—there is a third one: not to choose at all. Edmond Cahn defended this doctrine in terms of a dramatic tragedy, the overloaded lifeboat which will sink with all on board if some do not sacrifice themselves or are not put overboard either by drawing lots or by selection. Cahn's judgment was that all must live or die together, and like my guest, the dean of theology, that to choose is a demonic pretension. But this non-choice position has little to be said for it ethically compared to the alternatives. Choice by chance and choice by selection at least *try* to cope.

Choice-by-chance is a contradiction in terms. To resort to sortilege (a legal term for drawing lots) or casting dice or turning a card is, so to speak, a decision not to decide. It is a moral evasion of decision making and its anxieties, and as Kierkegaard said, "To venture is to become anxious, but not to venture is to lose oneself." It is irresponsible, a rejection of the burden. Its refusal to be rational is a deliberate dehumanization, reducing us to the level of *things* and blind chance.

The ethical issue at stake is plain enough, uncomfortably so. Are the needs of the one or the few subordinate to those of the many? Which prevails in actual conflicts, the common or the private interest? Let it be carefully noted, by the way, that to be impersonal in the sense of counting noses is not by any means to be antipersonal. It is multipersonal. If some of us cannot see the trees for the forest, others cannot see the forest for the trees. The point is this: To sacrifice the one for the many is to sacrifice the one for many *ones*. The "greatest number" is not an abstraction; it is the sum of real, particular, and personal individuals.

Hegel, in his short essay on logic, reasoned that the headachy business of choosing between one good and another, or obversely between one evil and another, is true tragedy, whereas the simplistic collision of good and evil—black and white—is only melodrama, Sunday School ethics. It is hard for Shakespeare's Othello to decide between his love of Desdemona and Iago's testimony, or for Sophocles' Antigone to choose between her loyalty to her brother and her loyalty to King Creon. So it is with all competing value problems. All serious ethics, as in a socially just health care system, deals with tragedy, not with melodrama—with choices between competing values, not with obvious matters of good and evil, right or wrong.

In the ethics of health care delivery we must be utilitarians, at least in the sense of seeking the greatest good (health) for the greatest number possible. Or, as Kenneth Boulding puts it, without counting and cost-benefit analysis "all evaluation is random selection by wild hunches." He adds, "The fundamental principle that we should count all costs, whether easily countable or not, and evaluate all rewards, however hard they are to evaluate, is one which emerges squarely out of economics and which is at least a preliminary guideline in the formation of the moral judgment, in what might be called the 'economic ethic.' "[7]

Just as people like Paul Samuelson and Robert Dorfman have coined the term "econometrics" for mathematics and quantification methods applied to economic data, I suggest that "ethimetrics" can be used for ethical analysis seeking distributive justice. It is a good label for applying statistical terms of amount and probability to macromoral problems, even down at such levels as allocating funds between developing an acceptable artificial heart and meeting the needs for patients in renal failure. To be ethical requires knowledge and careful calculation, because loving concern is the same as justice—it has to be distributed.

All of this leaves many loose ends and unopened boxes. The overall questions are, presumably, whether ethimetrics is (a) workable and (b) desirable. A great deal of thinking is called for, much of it new thinking, before we can catch sight of any consensual principles. Here are half a dozen worrisome questions:

1. Is it really necessary to weight values numerically, to quantify qualities? Why could we not just get the data numbers from the computers and then, with the factual data in hand, choose between the options thus measured according to our ranked but unquantified values? Some, like Toulmin, think the answer is yes, we can. Some would even contend that "quantifying quality" is impossible, a contradiction in terms.

Jay Forrester of the Massachusetts Institute of Technology once told me that a middle course is called for: first to program a computer's bank with all the data of macroethical questions, then to assign relative numerical weights to the values involved (a basically ethical, nonmathematical step) and enter them into the computer too, and finally to ask it to compute which course will yield the greatest human benefit.

2. Will distributive justice, if seriously pursued, homogenize quality or reduce it to mediocrity, reduce human valuations to a dead level, the least common denominator? In utilitarian theory there is a classic disagreement. Should we seek total or aggregate happiness—five million totally happy people or ten million moderately happy people? Should we aim at the most for some, or the average (aggregate) for all? Distributive justice seems to favor the aggregate principle, but am I right about this, and how shall we regard the issue's bearing on ethimetrics?

3. Is it the case, as ethicists of the school of emotive theory assert, that our values are inescapably subjective, in some degree personally arbitrary, even when shared widely with others? And even if they are, does this mean that a working consensus or common mind about what things are worthwhile, and in what order, is unreachable? If unreachable, what does this say about the claims of a democratic society? Does it and must it function without a common mind and common interests? Without consensus as its first premise, how can a legislature or government justify itself?

4. Given a consensus about "the good," or human happiness, is the proper business of a legislature or law-making body anything but or besides the utilitarian task, i.e., seeking the greatest good for the greatest number?

5. Is there really a persuasive case to be made, as some have always contended, for refusing to select and choose among human beings' needs, especially when human life is at stake? Or for resorting uncount-

ingly to sortilege when face to face with tragic choices and distributions? To take the stance that some things, whatever that covers, may not be done no matter how much good would follow, is obviously deontological—opposed to the teleological ethics of calculating benefits and consequences. It appears that the tactics of absolute rules are incompatible with the tactics of value optimization. Is this contradiction real? If so, can deontologists get around it somehow?

6. Surely all values do not have to be politicized, in the sense of socially distributed. Which ones should, which should not? And of those which should be, should they be distributed on the democratic one-man-one vote method, or what Garrett Hardin calls "mutual coercion mutually agreed upon"?[8] In democratic countries some values are usually excluded from the public dominion—tastes in music and the arts, for example. Furthermore, the logic of utilitarianism does not require the greatest good of the greatest number to be determined democratically, although almost all utilitarians in the West have been democratic for good reason.

An eminent bioethicist said to me recently, "It is time we began taking social medical ethics seriously." He is right, of course, but it is going to take lots of hard and novel thinking.

1. John Knowles, "The Unseen Ostrich in Our Teaching Hospitals," *Prism* 1 (November 1973), 13.

2. Hans Jonas, "Philosophical Reflections on Experimenting with Human Subjects," *Daedalus* 98 (Spring 1969), 238.

3. Daniel Callahan, *The Tyranny of Survival* (New York: The Macmillan Company, 1973), 184.

4. Albert Jonsen, "The Totally Implantable Artificial Heart," *The Hastings Center Report* 3 (November 1973), 5, 1-4.

5. Gordon Rattray Taylor, *The Biological Time Bomb* (New York: World Publishing Company, 1966), 211.

6. Roger Shinn and Warren Weaver, *Christianity and Crisis* 20 (January 23, 1961), 24, 210-15.

7. Kenneth Boulding, "Economics as a Moral Science," *The American Economic Review* 59 (March 1969), 7-8.

8. Garrett Hardin, *Exploring New Ethics for Survival* (New York: Viking Press, 1972), 128-32.

Five

Sharing with Others

The challenge of a just distribution or sharing of limited resources is posed with special appeal when we open our eyes, uncomfortably, to the hunger and starvation of millions of human beings in the world. Ethical analysis often goes deeper than ordinary social studies and reaches a fresh and startling viewpoint.

"Philosophers are back on the job," said Peter Singer recently, in a magazine piece about the revival of interest among philosophers in specific ethical problems.[1] He meant that the "wisdom lovers" are once more ready to examine more down-to-earth human problems than their once-fashionable "language analysis" permitted. Aristotle was right all along; politics is ethics writ large, and thus it is that the debate about helping the hungry, especially feeding them, is an excellent forum for showing what critical reasoning can accomplish.

Ethically regarded, famine relief is not a particularly complicated or knotty problem. As in everything else, any proposition about a person's or group's or country's obligation to help hungry or starving people has to satisfy three reasonable requirements: (1) that it is based on facts, data, evidence, (2) that it is logically consistent, and (3) that its foreseeable consequences are defensible. (These canons do not apply to astrology, for example, nor do they fit some philosophies of "sharing" either.)

The official foreign aid policy of the United States, as reflected in the literature and history of the United States Agency for International Development, stands on three legs—emergency aid, developmental assistance, and population control. This policy is, as we shall see, rationally acceptable, but it is acceptable *only if and when* qualified by an essential discrimination between needs arising from catastrophe or underdevelopment, as against needs arising from high fecundity and an irrational fertility rate. In some cases, we shall argue, population control should not only be encouraged but stoutly required as a condition or precondition of help.

Just as there are three requirements for valid obligation and three legs to American foreign aid, there are also three kinds of aid to be examined, compared and selected among. They are (1) *developmental assistance*, helping underdeveloped countries educationally and technically to accumulate capital and raise their standard of living, (2) *emergency famine or disaster relief*, as with earthquakes, floods, typhoons or atypical droughts—an instance being when a hurricane hit Honduras some years ago, and (3) *relief for countries suffering chronic famine* because their reproduction is excessive in relation to their actual or potential productivity. In this last case we ought not to help, it will be argued, until a workable and sincere commitment is made contractually to reduce such a country's fertility.

Religious activists, in a show of Jamesian tough-mindedness, have promoted undiscriminating feed-the-hungry programs. Their rhetoric reminds us, correctly enough, of such things as inequitable global distributions of food, equivocal government policies, big and exploitative agricultural corporations, and outrageous overconsumption (especially in America). However weighty, these are all sociopolitical factors. It says nothing about the basic, biological order, nothing ecological. Their appraisal never asks whether some countries have exceeded their carrying capacity by spawning more mouths to feed than the ecology allows.

I will contend that in at least a few cases certain countries have exceeded their biological carrying capacity, and that therefore to give them food is immoral. We often hear appeals to "the right to eat," but I shall reject any notion that rights are self-validating regardless of the relativities. Ethical analysis should determine right and wrong contextually or situationally, not by predetermined rules or moral imperatives; and in this modality both values and judgments, along with moral claims (rights), should be treated as variables according to the shifting factors within which ethical policies and decisions have to be shaped. Therefore, it could be right to send food or wrong to send it, depending on the situation and the foreseeable consequences. I shall also presuppose that we ought to seek the greatest possible good for the greatest number possible.

One relief crusade is "Food For Our Neighbors," a Billy James Hargis evangelistic program which solicits money to send food indiscriminately both to Bangladesh, a high-excess country, and to Mexico—a country which is thus far, at least, decidedly in biological balance. They explain that they work through missionaries (which reveals their ulterior motive), and their lack of ethical acumen is revealed in a typical appeal for "innocent children" with the injunction, "Pray, and let your heart rule your actions." It is boorish to knock prayer and we all admire plenty of heart and nobody wants children to suffer, but even if the motive of such appeals *were* disinterested, their concern for human beings is undermined by refusing to let their brains work.

Any suggestion that there are rational conditions for generosity sets the visceral functions of many people at war with their cerebral functions. What results is a high-flown but logically circular sentiment, "We ought to feed the hungry because they are hungry." A *circulus in probando* or *petitio principii* of this kind appears in the thinking of an economist in the Food and Agricultural Organization. Writing on the subject of feeding hungry peoples, he says, "It shall be done because it must be done."[2]

To ask seriously whether sharing will help or hurt shocks the superficial, who have never grasped how ethically wrong generosity can be. Such innocents are too easily dismissed by cynics—many of the latter being admirably hardheaded but deplorably hardhearted. To be situationally realistic about generosity by no means calls into question the virtue of generosity, as such. To ask, for example, what Americans ought to do for hungry Upper Voltans or Mauritanians is humane, not chauvinistic. Even if, arguably, charity begins at home, if it stops at the water's edge it withers into group-egoism.

If we want to ask analytic questions seriously, we should follow the advice of the mathematician Karl Jacobi; it was, "*Umkehren, immer umkehren*" ('invert, always invert').[3] We ought not go on asking, Who would be helped by our help? We need also to ask, Who would be *hurt* by our help? Relief is not always or necessarily helpful. This inversion strategem is a very useful tool ethically. By inverting we can see that in some situations we may actually hurt people if we send them food. In some instances even non-food assistance might at least be futile, if not hurtful. In situations where reproduction has outstripped productivity, to give food would only increase the population without raising the rate of production, thus increasing the number of starving people in a net loss of life and a net increase of human misery.

Sometimes we hear specious or at least secondary objections to sending food relief to famine areas—objections having to do with alleged or known misfeasance or even malfeasance in the distribution of relief, or doctrinaire and ideological protests, as in sales of grain to Russia or Poland, and the like. But these are not fundamental, when compared to objections based on biological-ecological limits and imbalances.

Somebody is sure to say, as a label and perhaps as an epithet, that to reason this way is Malthusian or neo-Malthusian. The latter term fits better, if the thesis has to be christened. We are frequently reminded by competent demographers, social biologists, climatologists, and geographers that we cannot feed everybody in the world. The thesis here, however, is that we *ought* not to feed everybody. It is therefore an ethical thesis, resting on the interface between population and the standard of living. Marx said that production and reproduction are the two basic realities of human existence, and Malthus (much earlier) saw that baby making can nullify the supposed benefits of wealth making. Both, thus far, were correct.

Malthus reasoned that population tends to increase faster, in a geometric ratio, than the means of production to provide food. Food, he held, increases only in arithmetic ratio. And, he went on, this will result in a chronic low supply of food *except* when war, famine, and disease reduce the population *or* it is checked by "sexual restraint" (meaning late marriage and continence.).[4] His "positive checks" on population (war, famine and disease) did not include contraceptive birth control because Malthus—a good eighteenth century clergyman—believed it to be immoral. (He was in much the same bind as the Pope still is today, recognizing the actuality of overpopulation but forbidden by a moral rule to act rationally.)

Neo-Malthusians take to heart the biological tension between population and wealth as mutually limiting factors, but they agree with William Godwin and Condorcet against Malthus that the best positive check on fertility is birth control rather than disease or war or famine. The Reverend Mr. Malthus was an economic pessimist who believed we would *always* be impoverished by fecundity; thus the new social biology shifts away also from his naturalistic pessimism to a trust in the workability of rational control. Also unlike Malthus, neo-Malthusians call for cutting down fertility, not for cutting out sex.

If a country of twenty-five million stomachs and an annual population increase of one million exceeds its carrying capacity and falls into chronic famine, with a vital balance of ten births and ten deaths annually per thousand, to give them food would prolong the progenitors' lives and in about twenty years they would double the population. At the established balance there would then be *two* million births and deaths per year; the quantum of human suffering would have been doubled in a net loss of lives to disease and starvation. Contrary to what some relief advocates say, this neo-Malthusian analysis does not assume that such countries will *never* lower their birth rates. It does assume, however, that if their birth rates are *not* lowered to a biological balance of people and environment, they cannot escape their predicament.

It may help this discussion along if we use "Third World" (by now a familiar label) to stand for underdeveloped countries like Indonesia. This grouping includes countries with national economies which have yet to achieve enough capital development and technological sophistication but nevertheless have a social-biological balance favorable to development. They have a favorable ratio among the five primary factors: population, pollution, raw materials, food supply, and industrial output. Given a sociobiological balance, development presents no great obstacles. At the close of World War II ninety percent of the world's countries were stagnant economically. Today fewer than half of them are in that class, due mainly to developmental assistance.

The term "Fourth World" has lately emerged as another category, representing undeveloped as distinguished from underdeveloped countries. The Fourth World consists of about 40 countries, countries whose standard of living is at the lowest level. Among these is a *small* (we may be thankful) category which exceeds its carrying capacity (too many people) and in consequence faces chronic famine plus a paralysis of capital growth. For this bottom-of-the-barrel group we should coin the name "Fifth World."

In this Fifth World group might go India, Bangladesh, Upper Volta, Senegal, Niger, and a few others. (This is a question for the requisite experts rather than for ethicists—deciding which countries are "Fifth.") In any case, they are unlike the Third and Fourth World countries because they are biologically stymied, without a rationally founded hope unless they reduce their population and reconstitute their soil—the source of their food and raw materials. In that struggle the affluent (developed countries) could help the impoverished by giving assistance (growth support), but the help should not be in the form of food shipments.

Assistance to the Fifth World would include seed capital and pilot equipment, which could be rented, sold, lent or given outright, along with technical, educational and medical training, to build their capabilities and increase the productivity of their labor. Even in such cases of assistance, however, we find a specialist such as James W. Howe, an able spokesman for United States Aid to International Development, qualifying his advocacy with a statement that "assistance would be of doubtful morality if it were absolutely certain that fertility could not be reduced over the decades ahead."[5] (Phrased in this way he could, in the recesses of his own mind, be quite unconditional about assistance since demographic projections cannot be "absolutely certain.")

Howe demonstrates the peculiar logic with which help-the-hungry advocates usually do their work. Having thus acknowledged that fertility is the key to successful aid, he then adds that "to assume a permanent inability to reduce births is to say there is no hope that these countries will ever escape the Malthusian dilemma." In truth, the assumption is just the opposite of what he suggests, namely, that if these countries do not escape the Malthusian dilemma by reducing their birth rates, there is no hope of their escaping from a situation where many are permanently hungry and starving.

Even if we take a global Spaceship Earth stance rather than a national economy Lifeboat stance, we ought not to feed Fifth World peoples who continue in their present reproductive mores. Even if we feel we ought to help Third and Fourth World countries (as I for one do), we ought not to send food to the countries which suffer from chronic famine no matter how saddened or upset we are by their plight. Undiscriminating generosity, fired by feelings of false guilt when comparing high standards of living to sub-subsistence, is appropriate only to "liberals" of the most sentimental kind. Our own wealth and ability to relieve hunger is morally irrelevant, whenever the consequence of feeding the starving is to make things worse in terms of human well being. Feeding the hungry in some countries only keeps them alive longer to produce more hungry bellies and disease and death.

Calling the United States and the Soviet Union "fat cat" countries which "ought to be ashamed to be so selfish" is pure ethical rubbish, sentimental and uncritical and therefore irresponsible, if the charge is made in blanket terms without careful use of the carrying capacity criterion. Garrett Hardin's challenge, in effect, is to ask us the searching question ethically—Do good intentions excuse the consequences of our actions? The Fifth World with its suffocating birth rates and depletion of its soil is deep in nihilistic immolation, and to become accessories after the fact is indefensible—if you have enough loving concern for human beings to want to minimize suffering. To minimize suffering is one important way of maximizing the good.

One school of thought about helping the world's poor offers what the unwary might take to be a way out of the neo-Malthusian dilemma. The dilemma is that famine relief helps excessive reproducers to survive and thus to increase the number of famine victims. The alleged way out of this is called the *demographic transition theory*. As a theory it is both debatable and in fact much debated. Its exponents argue that with capital development and a rise in the standards of living the rate of reproduction falls. This appears to have happened as a coincidence in some times and places, but it is not uniformly the case nor causally established. The evidence supporting it is more anecdotal than scientific. In the United States, to take a rich country, its enormous technical development has been paralleled by an enormous population *growth*, in the secular or overall trend.

This theory might influence some moral judgments about offers of help to Third and possible Fourth World countries, but if it ever applies at all to Fifth World countries it should only influence decisions to offer assistance, not food. One well-known American foundation regularly gives nearly four hundred thousand dollars in grants for an irrigation project in Niger, but not one cent for food. We should be asking invertly what Dives's generosity does to Lazarus, not only what it does to or for Dives and his spiritual brownie points.[6] Even as tough-minded a person as Robert McNamara, president of the World Bank, never asks the question—perhaps because it is inexpedient to raise it, and undiplomatic.

A typical instance of uncritical thinking about hunger in the world was illustrated by an Aspen Conference of Jews and Christians in 1974. Everybody there assumed we should aid *all* hungry people, apparently with priority going to the hungriest and most desperate, which is exactly the opposite of medical triage. They made no attempt to answer the neo-Malthusian thesis, contenting themselves moralistically and piously with the saying, "As you do it unto the least of these my brethren you do it unto me."[7] On the other hand, the World Development Council (which engineered the Aspen meeting and published its proceedings) quite aggressively confronts the neo-Malthusians by appealing to the demographic transition theory.

Be it noted, however, that the World Development Council's analysts *never ask whether there are some situations in which food should not be given.* They never invert. For the most part, their promotion of the assistance principle is entirely reasonable ethically. It is "development" that concerns them chiefly, not relief. But too much of their discussion is at fault ethically because it fails to appreciate and make use of the distinctions between developmental assistance, emergency aid, and chronic famine relief. The same complaint can be lodged against Oxford Famine Relief, a more militant organization which, like the Council, fails to make situational distinctions or allocations.

The 1974 international meetings in Romania and Rome (the former on population, the latter on food) provided a striking contrast in rationality. The food conference managed to be realistic and fairly candid. The population conference was a shambles of both reason and honesty. It was dominated by Third and Fourth World politicians and ideologues, and their line was an undiscriminating appeal to human rights—an

alleged right to eat and an alleged right to reproduce—motivated politically.

Their purple oratory appealed idealistically to an objective moral
order, preaching that we "ought" to feed the hungry just because they
are hungry, regardless of the situation or consequences. For them ethics
meant rights (claims), not responsibilities. They perpetrated unblushingly
the most simplistic ideas about feeding and breeding. Away from the
rostrum and its microphones, however, comments were muttered such as
"Groceries, yes, but not without vasectomies."

The point is that when help hurts the recipients by increasing the
number of sufferers, it is wrong to give it. The food exists, of course. In
1970 it would have taken only twelve billion tons of cereals to increase
the caloric intakes of 460 million sufferers from malnutrition by 250
calories each. This is about one percent of the world's consumption, less
than half of what Americans throw away, about 30 percent of what is fed
to livestock in the United States. The question is not *can* we feed the
hungry of Blankland, but *should* we. It is an ethical, not a technical
question.

Giving food to the countries most destitute and seemingly bent on
ecological suicide only deprives others that could benefit. The argument
that corrupt and elitist rulers in some lands prevent help from reaching
the needy is often enough true, on the record, but it is always a questionable assumption. Undemocratic or vicious governments sometimes
strengthen their hold by using donated food to feed the hungry. The
obverse, that by *not* feeding the starving we can undermine such governments, is not too likely. It is a mistake to suppose that the hungry and
desperate will organize a new regime; more often they fall to fighting
each other. Even if a bad government falls, there is no good reason to
expect its successor to be more just or benevolent. In any case, widespread hunger is only secondarily a political issue. Basically, it is a
problem in social biology.

The kernel of the question appears when we face a standard appeal
such as, "Look at how much of everything we have and how easily we
could feed the goat-herding people who are starving in the Sahel or sub-
Saharan Africa." (As little as 15 percent of the wheat grown in the
United States is enough to feed its own population well; Kansas alone
grows enough to do it.) Ethically examined, the kernel of the question is
that whether *we* are rich or poor, affluent or not, is irrelevant to the
issue. It is relevant only to ask whether sharing will help or hurt the
recipients.

(It is appropriate, also, to ask whether sharing will help or hurt the
donor as well. Assuming there is a moral gain in acts of constructive

generosity, it still remains necessary to find out at what point (1) our giving *hurts* us in the sense of making it a real or felt sacrifice, at what point beyond that (2) sharing becomes *dangerous* to the donor, and finally at what point (3) it would be self-destructive, suicidal. In another place, I have argued that we rich Americans should individually and collectively share where it will help, at least up to the first point where it hurts, and arguably sometimes up to the second point, danger, yet not to the suicidal point.[8] But this has to do with developmental assistance to Third and Fourth World countries, whereas the problem we are examining here is whether to send *food* relief for chronic famine in Fifth World countries.)

The world as a whole is hungrier today, has far more undernourished or actually starving people in it, than probably at any time since mankind generally (not simultaneously) passed over from nomadic to agrarian societies. In a few countries which have achieved a high level of technical development in agriculture as well as in industry, people consume food to the extent of overindulgence. The average American swallows twice as much protein as the human body can use, and the steers we eat are ridiculously inefficient converters of plant to animal protein (about one pound per twenty-one pounds of feed).

One engaging and earnest advocate of help for the hungry, working in disregard of the distinctions being drawn here, was annoyed because John Knowles, president of the Rockefeller Foundation, had said, "Malthus has already been proved correct." She retorted, "If our agricultural resources were used rationally and distributed at all equitably, there would be enough [in the whole world] to go around now."[9] The truth is that (1) the world's resources are not distributed equitably mainly because good soil and raw materials are not distributed equitably, (2) there are no global structures politically and economically to provide a supranational distribution, (3) national sovereignty prevents a world government which might limit the consumption of rich foods and scarce energy-fuels in affluent countries, and (4) a few countries which exceed their carrying capacity are acting most irrationally and lethally by their excessive reproduction.

This is the right point at which to speak bluntly to the anti-ethics of excessive reproduction. In Bangladesh, a typically irrational country in its death-dealing fertility, seven babies are born every minute in a land with fourteen hundred Bangladeshi per square mile. The Bangladesh peasant progenitors think their children are their only security against old age. But if only two out of five children survive (that is the actual situation), what they have done in every case is to doom three of their own children in order to better the parents' chance of not dying themselves. This is a ruthless numbers game, a parlay *en masse*, with human lives as chips—a gambling game of prodigal prolificity. It is reinforced by religious teachings about an alleged divine approval of it. In fact, of course, they are victimizing their own children for their own gain, as well as hurting their own countrymen collectively and any foreign "bene-factors" who might be sending them food.

Education and health care can hold down and reverse such fertility rates, as we have seen in Sri Lanka, Costa Rica, Egypt, Taiwan, and Barbados. If the excess population is not eliminated, helping the Fifth World countries is inhumane and therefore immoral, a band-aid treat-ment to cover up the real sore. The new post-1950 China is a large-scale instance of how a high-fertility ethos, centuries old, can be changed. Some Quakers now confess that the problem is not food but fertility: "If Quaker world relief were to make a dramatic and sustained shift in such a direction, we might again provide the model for a crucial change in humanitarian efforts everywhere, and later generations might indeed 'rise up and call us blessed'."[10]

When deciding which Fifth World countries we ought to help, it is ethically irrelevant to ask, Do I need large portions of meat? or Do I need meat and bread every day? or How else can I get enough proteins? Arranging "fasting meals" and "foodless banquets" may have some nutritional value for the overfed, but that is all. If such sentimentalities help people to perceive the problem, all right, but if they send food to the victims of chronic famine they are unethical.

Garrett Hardin embraces the act-utilitarian method of situation ethics. He expresses it in his own formulation, "The morality of an act is a function of the state of the system at the time the act is performed—this is the fundamental tenet of 'situation ethics'."[11] He takes killing an elephant as an example. Killing one this year might be moral, indeter-minate two years from now, and immoral in five years. It depends on the consequences, and the consequences are shaped by the situation. To give developmental assistance or food relief, either one, without reckoning the cause or without counting the cost, is irresponsible, i.e., unethical. It is simply untrue to say without reservation that "It is more blessed to give than to receive."

Therefore, it is merely sentimental to say we *can* or *could* help the starving. What counts is whether such help will really help. Often it will, sometimes it will not. And by the same token, to say we can or could lower the birth rate to make help effective is not good enough. We would have to say we *are* doing it, or we *have* done it.

Alan Berg of the World Bank has contended, "If it were not for aid there would be many more starving babies."[12] In flat contradiction we have to say that in some countries it would be *because* of aid that there are more starving babies. Alan Gregg, a past vice-president of the Rockefeller Foundation, saw the problem more clearly and described overpopulation as a cancer, adding that he had never heard of a cancer being cured by feeding it.

It all boils down to the formula, Give if it helps, not if it hurts.

1. Peter Singer, "Philosophers Are Back on the Job," *The New York Times Magazine,* July 7, 1974, 6-7, 17-20.

2. Robert C. Tetro, quoted in Thomas Y. Canby, "Can the World Feed Its People?" *National Geographic* 148:1 (1975) 31.

3. I am indebted to Garret Hardin for this; from "Carrying Capacity as an Ethical Concept," *Soundings* 69 (Spring, 1976).

4. Thomas Robert Malthus, *An Essay on the Principles of Population as It Affects the Future of Society, with remarks on the Speculations of Mr. Godwin, M. Condorcet, and Other Writers* (London: 1798).

5. James W. Howe and Staff of the World Development Council, *The U. S. and World Development: Agenda for Action in 1975* (New York: Praeger Paperbacks, 1975), 65.

6. This question is the one which was not sufficiently examined in Hardin's brilliant and much contested essays, "Lifeboat Ethics: The Case Against Helping the Poor," *Psychology Today* 8 (1974) 38-43, and "Living on a Lifeboat," *Bioscience* 25 (1974) 561-568.

7. Report of the Aspen Interreligious Consultation, *Global Justice and Development* (Washington, D.C.: Overseas Development Council, 1975).

8. See Joseph Fletcher, "Feeding the Hungry: An Ethical Appraisal," in *Lifeboat Ethics,* ed. G. R. Lucas and T. W. Ogletree (New York: Harper and Row, 1977), 52-69.

9. Frances Lappé, "Fantasies of Famine," *Harper's Magazine* 2:1497 (February 1975) 54.

10. R. B. Crowell, "Lifeboat Ethics and the Quaker Conscience," *Friends' Journal* 21 (May 1975) 294-296.

11. Garrett Hardin, *Exploring New Ethics for Survival* (New York: Viking Press, 1972), 134.

12. Quoted in Ward Greene, "Triage," *New York Times Magazine,* January 5, 1975, 9 ff.

Six

Wasting Human Bodies

Up to this point we have seen some of the reasons for being clear about values, realities, and decisions. We have also seen something of the rigors of ethical probing. The main purpose of this volume being, however, to probe into biomedical ethics in particular, it is time now to turn in that direction.

We have entered a new era medically, and therefore culturally i.e., morally and ideologically. There are many highly portentous "breakthroughs" in modern medicine, and one of them we can call the Spare Parts Program.

Surgery and medicine, in partnership with technology, can *transplant* tissue by a graft from one person to another, such as skin or bone and organs like a liver or a heart, and from one part to another in the same person, such as blood vessels or cartilage. They can *implant* artificial materials and machines, e.g., synthetic arteries and electronic cardiac pacemakers. And they can *supplant* tissue—for example, with synthetic and plastic heart valves, or with kidney machines which can carry on the work of hemodialysis without the natural organ altogether. A lot of this spare-parts, or *cyborg*, medicine is only in an early stage of success, but it is here.

In World War II they called it cannibalizing when they put together parts of damaged lorries to make up whole ones. This kind of reconstruction is now an accomplished part of medicine. Not very long ago we found a measure of gallow's humor in saying that a dead body or cadaver was worth about eighty-seven cents—for its residual chemicals. But now a body has become very valuable—indeed, supremely precious—in terms of its lifesaving values.

Too much of the time when we speak of our era as a technological one, we have only discerned its character. We haven't really grasped it yet. In the midst of knowledge and power explosions, it is easy to let the present turn a corner into the future when we are looking the other way; then we get left too far behind. As Marshall McLuhan says, we live in a "rear-view mirror." We are not even as quick as Alice in her looking glass. We think of new things retrospectively, speaking of radios as "wirelesses" and autos as "horseless carriages" and trains as "iron horses" and refrigerators as "ice boxes" and cinematography as "moving pictures."

As we shall see, we are caught in something of this same lag with respect to medicine, and the result is that we are being prodigally wasteful in our funerary practices and stupidly selfish in our use of vital organs while we live and even more so when we die. It may not be too much to say that very often so-called reverent or pious death ceremonies, solemn "rites of passage" in the language of Van Gennep and the anthropologists, are nothing more than acts of callous indifference, and that our dying nowadays (80 percent of it in hospitals, not at home) is followed through in complete and selfish disregard for the health and even the survival needs of the living. What follows will be an explication of this charge.

The problem arises because medicine needs more "spare parts" for transplantation than it can find, and the issue is a cultural-ethical one. Ought we not to donate the human parts and tissue needed to save or enhance lives, and to give social reinforcement to such donations, whether the donors are well or near to dying? Emerson (in *Gifts*) said, "The only gift is a portion of thyself." He spoke more truly then he knew; we can take him far more literally than he ever imagined.

The resistance to this new dimension of man's struggle against disease and death comes mainly from deep-seated feelings about the body. The sense of identity and recognition is largely somatic, especially for the simple-minded. Even though we suffer when we lose a part of our own flesh and bone, we don't lose our self-recognition; we know who we are no matter how maimed we may be. It is, therefore, probably somewhat easier psychologically to volunteer a part of one's self than it is for family or friends to dispose of one's body on their own initiative. There are many situations in which kidneys, for example, have been promised by a donor patient, but nevertheless after death the family refuses to allow it. It seems somehow to them to be destroying or hurting or degrading those who have "passed on." Add to this image-making the powerful guilt components in grief reactions, familiar to us all, and we have no great difficulty in understanding (though not necessarily condoning) such "blocks" in the way of ethical responsibility. (The legal position is often so unclear and the sensibilities so poignant that hospital officials and physicians have usually bowed to this obstructionism, often at the expense of the recipient patient's life.)

The popular tendency has always been to combine vitalistic and organismic notions in the feeling that *life* somehow depends on organic unity and integrity, and that therefore personal identity or the *soul* does too. Its typical language form is religious, commonly in terms of a belief in or longing for survival after death. Few if any religious doctrines of eternal life and personal survival hold that the person to be "saved" is essentially corporeal, but the hunch-feeling persists that the *body* is sacrosanct; it is a form of religious materialism or physicalism.[1] Western piety and folkways have commonly lost sight of Aristotle's warnings against this kind of materialism in his first full-dress defense of the notion, in *The Soul* and in *The Generation of Animals*, as far back as the middle of the fourth century B.C. Christians, for example, forget or ignore Saint Paul's emphatic declaration, "It is sown a physical body, it is raised a spiritual body."

It has been a long time since very many people explicitly and consciously believed in the resurrection of the body in a kind of naive, non-Pauline conception of the "raised body" as a physical or material levitation or ascension. But just beneath the surface many people still feel that to lose a limb or an organ or a cornea is to enter "whatever comes next'" halt, maimed and blind. In the period from the first to the sixth century many Christians, indeed the majority, believed that the "saved" would, in duplication of Jesus' resurrection and ascension, rise from the grave and go "up" into eternal life—usually *en masse* at the last trump. In spite of the word games played rather skillfully by theologians to keep "body" from being understood in the flesh sense, it has been so taken and in some sects still is.

In modern times we have seen a considerable decline of explicit belief in an afterlife. Among the Semitic religions, this has not much troubled Judaism, which is relatively unmetaphysical and without any developed speculation about personal survival after death, but it has changed the focus of Christian and Moslem attitudes toward a greater concern for this world. By a happy twist, when we recall the history of classical and orthodox beliefs, this loss of faith in heaven and the next world tends to enhance appreciation of human life and values. And the modern man's understanding of soul and identity, cut loose from an earnest faith in immortality, *should* logically free people from the feeling that their real selves depend upon their keeping their bodies intact for the future life beyond the grave. Combined with theological reinterpretations of *body*, this disappearance of orientation to eternity should make it easier to overcome fearful and defensive objections to donating spare parts.

The body taboo adversely affects not only transplants but medical knowledge and education. People not only fail or refuse to offer their organs to transplant surgery, they also withhold them from the medical schools. And even from autopsy. We all know the story of the "resurrectionists" or body snatchers in the early nineteenth century, who came into being because anatomists could not legally get bodies for dissection. They continued their macabre robberies of graves until somewhat more enlightened laws allowed unclaimed bodies from prisons and poorhouses to go to medical schools instead of potter's fields. (Statute law reflects the intelligence and morality of the lawmakers and, in a democracy, of the people in general.) The problem of supply is very, very far from solved.

In 1519 Pope Leo X denied Leonardo da Vinci admission to a Rome hospital to study anatomy because he had once engaged in dissection. It was not until 1737 that the practice received official papal endorsement, which was repeated recently by Pius XII in an allocution to eye specialists in May, 1956. But to this day rabbis and mullahs are divided in their opinions.

Even now, we in the West are not too far advanced from the state of mind which resulted in the killing of five people in a New York City riot in April, 1788, when a mob burned the Hospital Society's building because it housed an anatomy collection. It wanted "no fooling with human bodies," and this attitude hangs on.

In a recent year, seventy-four hundred cadavers were needed for optimum instruction in American medical schools, but outside of two thousand unclaimed bodies available from morgues or other public agencies, there were only six hundred available by bequest—in the whole United States. These served only one-third of the need. Welfare benefits for the aged or indigent, since the Second World War, have greatly reduced the supply from the poor-dead.

When a choice has to be made between dissection for study or autopsy for diagnosis, the schools give way, on the ground, reasonable enough, that diagnostic or medico-legal requirements come first. Even here, in autopsy procedure, the body taboo constantly undermines moral obligation and responsibility to society. While 1.8 million Americans die each year—four-fifths of them in hospitals, only one-fifth in homes—*only one in six* is autopsied in spite of medical insistence on it for the sake of critical and research inquiry. (The better the hospital, the more autopsies are done. In the Massachusetts General Hospital, for instance, seventy percent of the dead are autopsied. Pathologists and their staffs have an important role in good medicine.)

Religious obstacles continue to block the expression of ethical concern and modern humanitarianism. In April, 1967, Orthodox Jews attacked the Knesset and government, in Tel Aviv and Jerusalem, as a protest against the practice of autopsy. This was tied to Talmudic law requiring that corpses be buried on the day of death, a rule which has run into much conflict with coroners' proceedings because of the hasty interment. The moral law also forbids a priest (*kohen*) or his descendants to come within four cubits of a cadaver, or to be under the same roof with one.[2] Some 358 religious leaders, including the two chief rabbis, called for the repeal of a 1953 law which allowed autopsies when three physicians certified a need to determine the cause of death. Judges in rabbinical courts asked synagogues to add to the Yom Kippur liturgy, "Our Father, our King, repel the evil of autopsies." People began refusing to enter hospitals, afraid their bodies would be "violated" if they died.

Rigid and orthodox Jewish religious law forbids mutilation, unless it is necessary to save the patient's life, or possibly to investigate a mysterious plague. This is a serious obstruction to transplant medicine, donations to eye banks, and the like.

The rabbinate, however, has approved proponderantly of organ transplants on the principle of *pikuakh nefesh* ("*saving a life*"), which permits breaking moral laws if life is in danger. The Ashkenazic Chief Rabbi in Israel declared (August, 1968) that transplants are allowed to save living patients, but organs may not be stored. Roman Catholic moral philosophy took much the same position until quite recently. (As we often find in these matters of specific or concrete moral questions, there is no Protestant discussion on surgery, autopsy, and other mutilative procedures—not even on the ethics of transplant donation.) In just the past five years, under the pressure of the rapidly increasing practice of spare-parts medicine, we have seen a marked and welcome change in Catholic moral theology. As recently as May, 1956, nevertheless, Pius XII expressed a papal disapproval of any attempt to offer an ethical justification for *inter vivos* transplants, from one living person to another, or for mutilations of any kind for any reason at all except to save the patient's own life or health. But ten years later the weight of theological opinion was still against Pope Pius, and it still is. (It is interesting to compare the even development of Catholic opinion on this question to the ups and downs of its contraception controversy).

In 1944 B.J. Cunningham published his *Morality of Organic Transplantation*, the first full-dress Catholic moral defense of the procedure. It fluttered the dovecotes. A long-standing principle of Catholic moral theology, the principle of totality, holds that (as Aquinas put it) the whole is more important than its parts, and therefore a *diseased* part may be sacrificed to save the health or life of the whole body. But does this mean that one may only undergo organ excision (mutilation) for one's sake, not for another's? The answer had been, for a long time, yes.

Things began moving in this century. In 1899-1900 H. Noldin said that a voluntary offer of any tissue would be a "violation of the Fifth Commandment" and "intrinsically unlawful."[3] But in 1923 A. Vermeersch could, to the contrary, say it would be "licit and commendable, though not of obligation"—i.e., justifiable on grounds of charity and the unity of mankind, but not required in conscience. However, the question had as yet so little urgency that these opposed opinions were given in footnotes. Father Cunningham's treatise opened it fully, a whole decade before kidney transplants started on a significant scale.

The issue was over invasion of a person's totality or bodily integrity. It did not affect post mortem mutilations. As McFadden points out, there is no ethical objection to cremation, dissection, autopsy, embalming, or bone banks contributed to *after* death.[4] Canon law allows hospitals to dispose nonceremonially of amputated limbs, excised organs, and so on, although burial in "holy ground" is preferred. Nor is there any moral objection, then, to organ transplants post mortem or cadaveric; the objection only arises with ante mortem or *inter vivos* donations.

In the whole matter of transplants, however, Cunningham had rested the case for them on a theory of radical solidarism, or the oneness of human beings as the family of God. He reasoned from this base that to give an ovary or testicle (or graft therefrom, as in the Voronoff procedure), or to give a kidney or an eye or any other paired organ, is not only an act of charity or loving concern but actually self-serving in the sense that the recipient is only the other self, an alter ego. It was this thesis in moral theology, and its conclusion, which Pius XII rejected in 1956.

Once the papal view had been published, doubt and disagreement began to be expressed. The official opinion amounted to this: that one may morally save his own life or health but not his neighbor's! Healy interprets Pius to have meant that "mutilation is licit only when necessary for preserving the health of the whole body"—i.e., the individual's own body.[5] This was practically the language also of Pius XI, in his encyclical *Casti Connubii*, 1930. McFadden puts it in other words, that Pius meant one may not deliberately submit to mutilation "to help some other person or to assist Society."

As the Jesuit moralist Gerald Kelly once said, it may "come as a surprise" to hear that it is wrong when donors "have as their purpose the helping of others"—in short, that it is wrong to be a *living* donor.[6] Father Kelly could not accept it, nor can most Catholic theologians of this day. It is recognized that to give a singular organ, such as the heart, is suicide, and no Catholic moralist is willing (as yet) to defend that much sacrifice. But sharing paired organs, such as the kidneys, is another matter. McFadden, for one, defends donations *inter vivos* on the grounds that the principle of totality calls for *functional* integrity, not mere anatomical integrity. On this view we may rightly remove a healthy appendix because it has no vital function or purpose, and we may give up a kidney because one (or even a third of one) might be enough to preserve renal function. Only if donor nephrectomies are shown to impair a necessary function are they to be declared illicit. Healy takes the same stand, speaking of "substantial" integrity or totality, but meaning functional.

There is, on this basis, little or no reason to question the morality of cadaveric transplants, or of giving one's organs for that purpose by ante mortem testament. J. J. Lynch, S. J., sees no objections *per se* to a cadaveric transplant, although there might be objections *per accidens*—i.e., in a particular situation. He asks only that three rational preconditions be satisfied: 1) it is a necessary means of last resort, 2) there is a reasonable hope of substantial benefit, and 3) the medical and surgical teams are competent.[7] This applies also to kidneys, livers, endocrines, lungs, corneas, skin, bones, blood vessels—to all organs paired or unpaired, and to all kinds of human tissue. Our problem is not so much with the theologians as with inhibited or indifferent rank-and-file clergy and doctors who either do not know these things, or do not care, or will not bother to think about them or teach and lead the people they profess to serve.

The trap into which religious ethicists fall is, of course, their legalism. They adumbrate principles or universals as first premises for their syllogistic reasoning; and then as empirical experience undermines their generalizations and as situations change the context in which human values are to be served, they are paralyzed by these first premises, which they usually suppose to have some sort of divine authority. As Henry D. Aiken and others have pointed out, the more primitive or religious a culture or tradition is, the more legalistic or rigid its morality, and the more mature and sophisticated it is, the more elastic and situational its morality.[8] Anthropology has provided convincing data to support this.

It is often said in medical circles that these ethical problems are questions without answers. This is true in the sense that there are no completely reliable generalizations of a normative kind to dictate or pre-decide what we ought to do. We cannot universalize right and wrong, or make them absolute, however loyal we may be to such values as human well-being and response to need. Nevertheless, there *are* answers in the sense of responsible and reasonable decisions in particular cases, and this, along with the insights we gain by good question-asking, is all we can or need to have. This is medical responsibility.

Most of the experience in organ transplantation to date has come from kidney dialysis and replacement. It got off to a good start in 1954 with a transplant done by Dr. Murray, Dr. Merrill, and Dr. Harrison at Peter Bent Brigham Hospital in Boston. Up to that time the only spare-parts surgery, except for corneas, had been structural (e.g., bone and cartilage) or cosmetic (e.g., skin and hair), but now it had reached the level of vital life-or-death functions.

At first the kidneys were isografts, i.e., from related donors *inter vivos*. In fact, because of the problem of rejection or "immune reaction," twins were the most promising donors and recipients. But gradually allografts (from unrelated donors) have been successful as immunosuppressive methods have improved, to the point that by now there is a much higher rate of success, coming close to 50-50. *Kidneys from living donors*, compared to cadaver kidneys, require fewer dialyses prior to transplantation, fail less often to "start," and have fewer rejection crises, and only half as many recipients have to be rehospitalized.

Helped by surgical experience, compatibility testing, and better immunosuppression, transplantation has moved from twin donors to related donors to unrelated donors, and from living to cadaveric transfers. Cadaveric transplants from unrelated donors allow for *two* kidneys, not just one. A cadaver pancreas has been stitched to the recipient's old and failing one; if it rejects, they can snip it off and all is as before. An auto fatality yielded a heart to one patient and a kidney to another; following a suicide, the heart and both kidneys and the pancreas were transplanted. Meanwhile, the great majority of renal-failure patients remain on hemodialysis machines, hooked to and dependent upon them either chronically or continuously, often at discouragingly great expense and inconvenience, even though dialysis is not desired by physicians or their patients, because of a lack of donors—both living and post mortem.

The first kidney transplants were called immoral or premature, as the Wright brothers were at Kitty Hawk. The same was said of Harvey Cushing's intercranial surgery, and of open-heart techniques in thoracic surgery. At the focal point of debate right now are heart transplants, evoking fear and reaction. The medical authority in the Soviet Union (Boris Petrovsky, Minister of Health), for example, once prohibited heart transplants until the rejection mechanism had been conquered. But in some of these failures of organ function, such as the heart's, to do nothing means odds of 100 percent against the patient, whereas to go ahead offers even at this stage a 40 percent chance of rescue in some cases (kidneys) and 20-40 percent in hearts.

No significantly different ethical questions are posed by other forms of spare-parts medicine such as endocrines, lungs and livers, or by non-organic transplants or grafts such as blood, blood vessels (arteries and veins), bones, cartilage, and corneas. A thymus from a thirteen-week-old girl was flown from London in a cold saline solution, and transplanted to a seven-month-old boy.

Even when there is no irrational objection to making a donation of tissue and organs, i.e., even though it is not looked upon as intrinsically evil or undesirable, there are still occasional or situational moral questions involved extrinsically. Let us look now at four of these questions which can easily be raised even by those who are willing, everything else being equal, to contribute spare parts. They are: (1) the risks entailed, (2) the problem of competent consent, (3) the principles of selection, given the scarcity or low supply problem, and (4) the ethical status of xenografts from animals, or interspecific organs and tissue. (This fourth one is really a pseudo-ethical question, but it merits a brief mention. It is pseudo-ethical because it judges values not by their functional or effective nature (consequences), but by some assigned inherent or "intrinsic" feelings about their "nature" regardless of consequences. Thus: "It is just *wrong* to put something from a pig into a person; I just *know* it.")

As for the risks taken, they can be both psychological and physical. In *inter vivos* transplants of kidneys, for example, the donor reduces his renal survival potential by half (but not his functional powers), and this might become a source of anxiety. If the donor is related to the recipient, the motive might be guilt compulsion rather than true loving concern, and thus result in delayed reactions or too late regrets. A recipient or donor may unconsciously not want to "share spares" with the other, and end up with destructive hostility feelings.

The physical risks are not very great. Wives or husbands often object to their spouses' "cutting down their survival chances" for a third person's sake, fearful for themselves or their dependents. Actually, if the donor subsequently develops the same organic failure he can be "rescued" too, in his turn. And the risk in the operation is very slight. Suturing in dogs is more difficult than in humans, yet hundreds are sutured successfully. Replantation, as of a severed hand, is more exacting than organ transplantation, and open-heart surgery is more difficult than heart transplants. After all, the risk rate in everything is always finite, and cannot be reduced to zero; even in general anaesthesia it remains at

1:1,500. Dr. George Reed of New York University once questioned whether, when sound criteria are applied and calculations of loss-gain made, we have a moral right *not* to try a transplant, or to be a donor.

The danger of rejection after transplantation is always a part of the situation. The antigens are built genetically right into the cell nuclei. Blood typing, quite apart from the "throwing" problem, eliminates about fifty percent of prospective donors in a given case, with about ten percent of available donors being compatible. This is a fact about transplantation which underlies the crucial importance of a wide choice of living or cadaveric donors being available. Progress in immunosuppression has been steady. One interesting line of inquiry has been suggested by the fact that mothers usually do not reject the fetus for nine months even though it is alien tissue. (Some speculate that the key is to be found in the placenta.)

Consent is a consideration in all medicine, especially in surgery and clinical experimentation. But it takes on an added dimension in matters of tissue donation. "Competent" consent legally and ethically is a matter of free choice (noncoercive and voluntary) and understanding of what is at stake ("informed"). Treatises on the subject follow an almost conventional pattern. For example, sometimes moralists decide that prisoners in penitentiaries are in the very nature of their situation not really free to be voluntary donors. Sometimes they say that patients are so influenced by physicians, even when the physician leans over backwards not to influence the patient, that they will make donations because "Doctor seems to want it"—not because they themselves do.

In almost any medical situation the patient will be able to understand only a part of what the facts and the probabilities are. Thus, competent consent should not be understood in an ideal or perfectionist way which makes it practically impossible. There will never be a fully competent consent given: while it should never be perfunctory, it will always have to be substantial rather than perfect, on any model.

The principles of selection to be followed are under debate. Shall machines or organs go to the sickest, or to the one with most promise of recovery; on a first come, first served basis; to the most "valuable" patient (based on wealth, education, position, what?); to the ones with the most dependents; to women and children first; to those who can pay; to whom? Or should lots be cast, impersonally and uncritically? Can we get away from questions of counterproductivity and cost-effectiveness? If we don't think people ought to be making such dread decisions about other people, should we not be calling from the housetops for more donors?

In Leeds, England, three aortic valves from a pig's heart were used in a thirty-eight-year-old mother's heart, quite successfully. One patient lived over nine and a half months on a chimpanzee's kidney. An ape's heart valves were used in a seventeen-year-old young man in Budapest in 1968. A pig's liver was used in Johannesburg for a forty-seven-year-old woman, but not transplanted; it was used outside her body, to perfuse her blood, and at once it brought her out of coma. Any objection to the practice must be based on irrational or arational sentiment; it is, indeed, only a pseudo-problem. For those who are thus prejudiced it is enough simply to point out that they had better be more vigorous in recruiting donors! More progress is being made in mechanical hemodialysis, for example, which is only a holding maneuver for patients, than in getting *people* to help people. We can build machines more easily than we can rally donors to help their fellow men. This is a *real* ethical problem. Who has a right to complain about xeno-grafts, if he has not offered to help by sharing human parts?

The crucial question—how are we to understand death?—obviously has a bearing on the problem of an adequate supply of human tissue. The fear that timid people have, that transplanters may redefine death in order to hasten the donor's death in terminal decline, results from pressures caused by the lack of organs—although the objectors rarely acknowledge what the obstacle is. Brain death calls for waiting twenty-four hours or so and a reconfirmed flat electroencephalograph reading. But a cadaveric heart has to be used sooner than that, unless put on a machine. For kidneys, twenty-eight hours is thus far the longest interim period between the donor's death and transplant before ischemia, the stoppage of blood flow and consequent anemia, ruins the tissue.

Dr. Cooley, who has supervised more heart transplants than any other surgeon, and with a higher proportion of survival success than anybody else, put it this way: "The heart has always been a special organ. It has been considered the seat of the soul, the source of courage. But I look upon the heart only as a pump, a servant of the brain. Once the brain is gone, the heart becomes unemployed. Then we must find it other employment."[9] At a grand rounds in March, 1968, I heard him say, "When the brain is gone there is no point in keeping anything else going."

This is, of course, the classical view of life or the soul (*psyche*) in the Western doctrine of man, a rational view reflected in, for example, a great deal of Catholic philosophy. We can hark back to Byron's lines, "Maid of Athens, ere we part, give O give me back my heart," and a witty critic's remark that the Greeks thought the liver and not the heart was the seat of the "soul" or person. He therefore proposed a paraphrase of Byron, "Maid of Athens, ere we sever, give O give me back my liver." Now it is time for a second paraphrase, in the light of modern medicine: "Maid of Athens, ere we're twain, give O give me back my brain." It is the encephalograph, not the cardiograph, which tells us whether "anybody is there" or not.

Much of the pressure behind new proposals for a cerebral definition of "brain death" (irreversible coma) comes from the time factor. "Functional death" is a new concept emerging because artificial methods can keep hearts or livers or kidneys going in comatose patients after the brain has quit. This maintenance is necessary so that cadaveric transplant organs can remain in "health" until they are excised and transferred to the recipient patient. The donor is not alive in any meaningful sense.

All will hang, of course, on what we mean by "a dying person" and it is high time we faced up to it. The conventional wisdom holds that we may not "hasten" a donor's death, but what is it to hasten death when we have methods now that both suspend death and reanimate after it? And in any case, surely it is ethical to speed dying up, once the donor is *in terminus,* if he has foreseen such a situation and consented not only to the transplant but to the speeding up.

The present jumble of state laws incited a meeting (in Philadelphia, July, 1968) of medical and legal specialists to draft a "uniform anatomical gift act." Most states have adopted general gift statutes to guarantee that the deceased's gift will not be denied by next of kin. But they all vary in important respects. Next of kin have been the moral bottleneck in Anglo-American law ever since the temporal courts threw out the church's probate jurisdiction over bodies (a change that took place in the late eighteenth century). A uniform law would help to protect physicians from next of kin trouble, since body taboo is still tragically persistent.

The big relief will come when human beings are no longer needed to help human beings, either by ante or post mortem help. The fact is that more progress is being made in devising artificial ways to save life than in getting human help with spare parts. But it is also true that there is greater promise of spare parts from animals than from humans. Just as herds of horses are specially raised for steaks on many luncheon tables (the Harvard faculty club's, for one), so herds of baboons and gibbons and cows and swine will be raised specially for tissue and organs transplantable into humans. Bio-engineers doing polymerization for chemically constructed tissue and electronic engineers devising organ substitutes, as well as dumb animals, can be counted on, in ways human beings cannot be counted upon, to help people caught in serious tissue loss and organic failure.

The use of interspecific material, however—and the use of human tissue too—will be greatly enhanced as the methods of preservation are worked out. It is not feasible yet to "bank" material for any length of time by freezing or hypothermia, since water in cell tissue expands on freezing and ruptures the membranes. Perhaps an antifreeze substance like glycerol will solve it. (In the Navy's center at Bethesda, Maryland, organs are being attached to baboons to keep the transplants going until the recipient is ready. And polio vaccine now is developed in monkey tissue.)

Continuous storage by freezing or perfusion is not solved for whole organs, and it is possible only for a few weeks even with skin, sperm, and vessels. It is easier, of course, for bone, cartilage and corneas. Successful animal experiments were reported recently which show that human organs could be stored as long as seventy-two hours, and indefinite freezing may be about a decade away. Machines can lengthen the time of preservation and expedite shipping interstate or cross-country. It is *this* kind of thing which medicine is counting on, not human generosity.

The troglodyte and "rear-view mirror" reaction to all this is, "You are playing God." Perhaps we should simply accept this description of what it means to use our new controls over life and death in a responsible way. The real question is *which* God we are playing when we shoulder the solemn and often perplexing burden of making vital decisions. It is "the God of the gaps," as theologians say, whose role and prerogatives we are preempting. This God is a hypothesis of ignorance, the honor we pay to what we do not know or cannot do, born and projected out of our feelings of awe and fear of the unknown—the *mysterium tremendum*. As we have learned and succeeded, that God has diminished and died. The God of the gaps is dead.

This is not a human or demonic pretension. On the contrary, the advance of our medical powers serves a humble and serious concern to be responsible, to respond to need effectively. Less and less do people die or suffer stupidly and helplessly, trapped in a value-blind "nature." Man's intelligence transcends nature progressively. And we might note that nothing is won by moderate counsel to go slow in our conquest of illness and death. The errors of moderate opinion are often harder to detect than those of extreme opinion, and for that reason they are often far worse and more dangerous, and certainly more likely to disarm us.

Every ill person, if free to choose life or a chance for it *in articulo mortis*, ought to be free likewise to choose *not* to go on living or to be brought back by resuscitation and transplant. On the other hand, he has less freedom or right, ethically, to refuse such a chance for others—for example, by giving his body or tissue.

The Convocation of Canterbury, Church of England, has voted to provide "pastoral guidance to those who bequeath their bodies for research or who wish parts of them to be available for transplants, and to those who have to make funeral arrangements when such use is made of their bodies." The day is coming, we may hope, when memorial services will take the place of selfish and unethical religious burial ceremonies.

1. Joseph Fletcher, *Morals and Medicine* (Boston: Beacon Press, 1961), esp. chaps. 5, 7.

2. Solomon B. Freehof, *A Treasury of Responsa* (Philadelphia: Jewish Publication Society of America, 1962), 236-241.

3. *Theologia Moralis*, II, 328n.

4. Charles J. McFadden, OSA: *Medical Ethics* (Philadelphia: F. A. Davis Co., 1961), 265-266.

5. E.J. Healy, SJ, *Medical Ethics* (Chicago: Loyola University Press, 1956), 122.

6. Gerald Kelly, SJ, *Medico-Moral Problems* (St. Louis: Catholic Hospital Association, 1958), 246.

7. J.J. Lynch, SJ, "Human Transplantation: A Theological Observation," *Linacre Quarterly* 35: 2 (May 1968), 122-125.

8. Henry David Aiken, *Reason and Conduct* (New York: Alfred A. Knopf, Inc., 1962), 116-127.

9. *Life*, August 2, 1968.

at it, a Canadian biologist, N. J. Berill, says, "Sooner or later one human society or another will launch out on this adventure, whether the rest of mankind approves or not. If this happens, and a superior race emerges with greater intelligence and longer lives, how will these people look upon those who are lagging behind? One thing is certain: they, not we, will be the heirs to the future, and they will assume control."[2]

Among religionists, Canon Michael Hamilton, of the National Cathedral in Washington, approves of genetic engineering, when and if it is aimed at the personal improvement of humans.[3] At the same time a Jesuit theologian, Richard McCormick, condemns it because, he believes, only monogamously married heterosexual reproduction is morally licit.[4] Wearing his philosopher's hat, J. B. S. Haldane votes for genetic design,[5] but putting on the same hat, another biologist, Theodosius Dobshansky, votes against it.[6] Disagreement is obviously at work at all levels and in all intellectual camps, from the simplest people to scientific peers.

A careful approach to the issue will avoid what I call the 'capacity-fallacy'—i.e., the notion that because we can do something, such as genetic control, we ought to. It does not follow that because we could, we should. There is an ethical parallel in the 'necessity-fallacy,' the assumption by some culture analysts that because we can do something, we will. Those who are fatalists—a visceral or noncephalic disposition that is fairly widespread among us—naturally do not bother to ask policy questions.

Leaving aside technical philosophical conventions, when we tackle right-wrong or good-evil or desirable-undesirable questions there are fundamentally two alternative lines of approach. The first one supposes that whether any act or course of action is right or wrong depends on its consequences. The second approach supposes that our actions are right or wrong according to whether they comply with general moral principles or prefabricated rules of conduct. Kant's formula, "It is always wrong to treat people as means and not as ends," would be an example of decision by moral rules, like the pacifist's use of the fifth of the Ten Commandments, "Thou shalt not kill." The first approach is consequentialist; the second is *a priori*.

This is the rock-bottom issue, and it is also (I want to suggest) the definitive question in the ethical analysis of genetic control. Are we to reason from general propositions and universals, or are we to reason from empirical data, variable situations, and human values? Which? One or the other.

Until modern times the most common form of *a priori* ethics was religious morality. It usually held in advance of any concrete or actual problem of conscience that certain kinds of acts, such as lying and stealing and fornicating, are always wrong intrinsically, in and of themselves, as such. Their inherent wrongness was believed by faith and by metaphysical opinion to be a matter of "natural" moral law or of divine revelation. They were always negatives, never affirmatives—prohibitions, not obligations. Such "moral laws" were presumably known to the moral agent—the actor or decision maker—through inner guidance or intuition, or by spirit guidance from outside, or by means of some more objective special revelation, like scriptures. In any case, right and wrong were determined by a religious or metaphysical or nonempirical kind of cognition. There is still a widespread disposition to take an ethical posture of this kind, even though it is often unconscious. It is metarational ethics.

Nonconsequentialists would say, therefore, that therapeutic or corrective goals are not enough to justify *in vitro* fertilization, positive eugenics, or designed genetic changes, no matter how desirable they might be. It was this kind of ethics that Daniele Petrucci ran into several years ago in Bologna because of his experiments with artificial fertilization and cell divisions at preblastocyst stages. The Church forced him to stop, in a kind of modern Galileo episode.

The basic moral law here was the religious belief that "only God can make a tree" and only God should make a man. On this basis it would be wrong to use artificial fertilization, insemination, or innovulation, or single cell replications in ectogenesis. This "law" of the divine monopoly is also opposed to any human control of sexually produced conceptuses. In the same way it is believed that the mere fact of fertilization results directly in a truly *human* being or at least a *nascent* human being, so that the laboratory sacrifice of such zygotes, or the use of a prostaglandin, being abortifacient, would be intrinsically wrong—i.e., "murder."

Good consequences could not, to the *a priori* moralist, justify such acts or procedures, since they are wrong as means, and the *a priorist* contends that the end does not justify the means. The principle of proportionate good, or a balance of gains over costs, could not in their ethics make genetic intervention by laboratory reproduction morally permissible. Consequences, as they see it, do not decide what is right. At a discussion at Airlie House, Dr. Leon Kass, a molecular biologist working for the National Research Council, put the *a priori* position succinctly. "Morally," he said, "it is insufficient that your motives are good, that your ends are unobjectionable, that you do the procedure 'lovingly' and even that you may be lucky in the result: you will be engaging in an unethical experiment upon a human subject."[7] This is also the opinion of

Paul Ramsey, a Protestant moralist who, like Father McCormick, believes that such procedures as artificial insemination from a donor, artificial innovulation, cloning, and other forms of asexual reproduction are wrong—wrong because morally licit reproduction must be done heterosexually by human intercourse within the context of marriage and the family.[8]

However, some *a priori* moral principles are not based on metaphysical grounds. One school of utilitarians, called 'rule utilitarians,' make moral choices on the basis of generalizations reached empirically or clinically. They might conclude that in the expectable results of laboratory reproduction and genetic engineering, the good would be outweighed by the evil, or that the attendant risks are unknown or too great, and that therefore such procedures should be disapproved as a class or category.

Rule utilitarians make no attempt to assign an intrinsic value or dys-value. Their reason for resorting to categorical principles is usually like G. E. Moore's: that they are unwilling to trust their own judgment in situations that are apparently exceptions to the general rule. They might therefore simply rule out some class actions (such as genetic designing) universally and categorically. Or again they might not. Outside some theological and philosophical circles, most of the opposition to designed genetic changes in man, or even to genetic intervention for therapeutic purposes, is based on rule-utilitarianism.

In this connection, by the way, it is only fair to point out that all religionists are not *a prioristic*. For example, Professor James Gustafson, of the Chicago Divinity School, has asked if biomedical changes in man are intrinsically wrong and answered in the negative, but he then added that if its consequences were antihuman it would for *that* reason be wrong.[9] (Later, we shall have cause to return to this matter of the human and nonhuman.)

The more commonly held ethical approach lies in a different modality, a pragmatic one—sometimes sneered at by *a priorists* and called a "mere morality of goals." This goal ethic is my own, and I believe it is implicit in the ethics of all biomedical research and development, as well as in medical care. We reason from the data of each actual case or problem and then choose the course that offers an optimum or maximum of desirable consequences.

On this basis we cannot reason deductively from *a priori* or predetermined rules about the moral justifiability of whole classes of acts, such as the *in vitro* fertilization of gametes and the experimental sacrifice of test zygotes, or the cloning of animal and human organisms. We agree with

Jeremy Bentham: "If any act can with propriety be termed pernicious, it must be so by virtue of some events which are its consequences...no act, strictly speaking, can be evil in itself."[10]

For those whom we might call situational or clinical consequentialists, results are what count, and results are good when they contribute to human well-being. On that basis the real issue ethically is whether genetic change in man will, in its foreseeable or predictable results, add to or take away from human welfare. We do not act by *a priori* categorical rules nor by dogmatic principles, such as the religious proposition that genetic intervention is forbidden to human initiative, or the metaphysical claim that every individual has an inalienable right to a unique genotype—presumably according to however chance and the general gene pool might happen to constitute it. For consequentialists, making decisions empirically is the sensible procedure. The question becomes, When would it be right, and when would it be wrong?

What, then, might be a situation in which constructive or positive eugenics would be justified because the good to be gained—the proportionate good—would be great enough? Another way of putting it is, When would its utility justify it? I am not much of a seer or forecaster, and I feel uncomfortable attempting to predict shocks of the future in long time-spans. But we have to try, even though trying it raises our anxiety level. We owe a great obligation to the future and to our descendants, and it would be irresponsible to repudiate the problem of genetic control by either a blanket condemnation or an uncritical endorsement.

Take cloning of humans, for example, as a form of genetic engineering. Although Joshua Lederberg, another Nobelist in microbiology, may be correct when he says that cloning is "merely speculative" until more experimental work with animals is done, it is still possible that such science fiction "scenarios" can help value analysis and ethical examination. Diderot, G. B. Shaw, H. G. Wells, Huxley, and Lederberg himself have all predicted genetic engineering. As crystal-ball gazers they have, until recently, been like Priam's daughter Cassandra, doubted and poohpoohed. But now things are different. Now not only the doomsday people but the tut-tut reactors are having a harder time.

And yet, just because cloning is defensible in asparagus or carrot growing, it does not follow that it is all right in human baby making. I respect the ethics of scientists, which is primarily a love of and search for the facts, but some scientists seem to have an almost blind faith that somehow the facts will be used to good purposes, not misused for evil. This is too complacent as we face the wide margin of personal and social dangers in biomedical research and practice. Therefore, whether and when genetic control could be right would depend on the situation. Let's look at a few cases, both therapeutic and eugenic.

There might be a need in the social order at large for one or more persons specially constituted genetically to survive long periods outside space capsules at great heights. Control of a child's sex by cloning, to avoid any one of fifty sex-linked genetic diseases, or to meet the imperatives of a family's survival, might be justifiable. I would vote for laboratory fertilization from donors to give a child to an infertile pair of spouses.

It is entirely possible, given our present increasing pollution of the human gene pool through uncontrolled sexual reproduction, that we might have to replicate healthy people to compensate for the spread of genetic diseases and to elevate the plus factors available in ordinary reproduction. It could easily come about that overpopulation would force us to put a stop to general fecundity, and then, to avoid discrimination, to resort to laboratory reproduction from unidentified cell sources. If we had "cell banks" in which the tissue of a species of wildlife in danger of extinction could be stored for replication, we could do the same for the sake of endangered humans, such as the Hairy Ainu in northern Japan or certain strains of Romany gypsies.

If the greatest good of the greatest number (i.e., the social good) were served by it, it would be justifiable not only to specialize the capacities of people by cloning or by constructive genetic engineering, but also to bio-engineer or bio-design parahumans or "modified men"—as chimeras (part animal) or cyborg-androids (part prosthetes). I would vote for cloning top-grade soldiers and scientists, or for supplying them through other genetic means, if they were needed to offset an elitist or tyrannical power plot by other cloners—a truly science-fiction situation, but imaginable. I suspect I would favor making and using man-machine hybrids rather than genetically designed people for dull, unrewarding, or dangerous roles needed nonetheless for the community's welfare—perhaps the testing of suspected pollution areas or the investigation of threatening volcanos or snow-slides.

Ours is a Promethean situation. We cannot clearly see what the promises and the dangers are. Both are there, in the biomedical potential. Much of the scare mongering by whole-hog or *a priori* opponents of genetic control link it with tyranny. This is false and misleading. Their propaganda line supposes, for one thing, that a cloned person would be a carbon copy of his single-cell parent because the genotype is repeated, as if such genetically designed individuals would have no individuating personal histories or variable environments. Personalities are not shaped by genotypes alone.

Furthermore, they presume that society will be a dictatorship and that such designed or cloned people would not be allowed to marry or reproduce from the social gene pool, nor be free to choose roles and functions other than the ones for which they had a special constitutional capability. But is this realistic? Is it not, actually, a mood or attitudinal posture rather than a rational view of the question?

Dr. Lederberg has pointed out that although the scenario of the Brave New World has been widely advertised, emphasizing that a slave state could and probably would use genetic control, still "it could not be so without having instituted slavery in the first place." He adds, "It is indeed true that I might fear the control of my behavior through electrical impulses directed into my brain but. . . I do not accept the implantation of the electrodes except at the point of a gun: the gun is the problem."[11] I agree. The danger of tyranny is a real danger. But genetic controls do not lead to dictatorship—if there is any cause-and-effect relation between them it is the other way around—the reverse. People who appeal to Brave New World and 1984 and Fahrenheit 451 forget this, that the tyranny is set up first and *then* genetic controls are employed. The problem of misuse is political, not biological.

The possibility of an ethical justification of genetic control, such as I have indicated, leads at once to the question of an ethical defense of its essential prerequisite—embryologic and genetic research. As I said at the outset, there are serious challenges not only to the end being sought (control) but also to the morality of the means—*in vitro* fertilizations, bench-made zygotes and embryos, and the entailed practice of their sacrifice in the course of investigation. If we can justify the end, can we justify the means? Does the end justify the means in this particular case? My answer is a positive yes.

I can see only one possible objection to such research, given a humanistic and situational ethics of the sort I have indicated. That objection would be that fertilizations or cloning would result directly and instantly in human beings, or in creatures with nascent or proto-human status. Let me say at once that I do not believe this to be true. And that is what such a proposition calls for—belief in a faith assertion, a declaration or confession of faith. It is not in the order of either scientific or rational statements to say that such early cell tissue is human (except in the sense of the biologic specification): it is an *a priori* metarational opinion. It effectively excludes from its ethics all nonbelievers.

For example, a Catholic obstetrician in Washington, D.C., has complained that it is "arbitrary" to start regarding a fetus as human at the twentieth week or at "viability," and yet the physician himself insists on the even more arbitrary religious doctrine that a fertilized ovum before implantation is human.[12] Granted that it is difficult to check off any specific point on the gestational continuum as the start of a human being, it is obvious that there is much more to be said for viability at that point than at the instant of fertilization.

Those who believe such things may be correct. There is no way to know whether they are or not. It follows for them deductively that abortion is wrong in any of its manifold forms, before or after nidation. It would also follow that the experimental sacrifice of zygotes and blastular embryos in the research process is the destruction of innocent human life or the "killing of unborn babies."

This rhetoric is again an instance of how *a priori* ethics reasons syllogistically from metaphysical and metarational premises to a normative conclusion, rather than reasoning consequentially. All the good results in the world, immediately or potentially, could not (they argue) justify what is wrong—in this case, "homicide." Indeed, if anybody really believes that a zygote is a human being, he or she ought not to terminate a pregnancy or engage in embryologic research, not only for the sake of ethical consistency, but for the sake of their own mental and emotional balance.

But most of us do not make that faith assertion. This is precisely and basically what is at stake in the national debate about abortion laws—the fact that they rest on grounds of a private, personal, religious conviction and should not therefore be established by government in violation of the Constitution's First Amendment. Obstetricians and gynecologists do not believe this doctrine, nor do surgeons, nor do fetologists, nor do embryologists and geneticists—except for an atypical minority involved with certain religious groups.

There are, be it noted, additional auxiliary arguments used sometimes against the research sacrifice of embryos and other fetal life, such as the claim that it tends to lower respect for human life. But this begs the question and is not really very convincing as a consequentialist argument (which it is, by the way). It is very likely in any case to be a cover-up for the notion that fallopian and uterine cell matter is human. There is also a "feeling" in some discussants that a conceptus somehow has a right to be born. They would be better advised to follow the reasoning of our common and statutory law, which rejects any idea of "unborn babies" and restricts the status of "baby" to the neonate, denying that any rights at all may be assigned to a fetus.

Nevertheless, these objections to laboratory reproduction uncover two further points I feel obliged to establish. Both points are metaethical in nature, or at least prenormative. The first has to do with the idea of *humanness* and the second has to do with the notion of *rights*.

What does it mean to say, as Dr. Kass does, that "the laboratory reproduction of human beings is no longer human procreation"? (Indeed, can he reasonably charge that laboratory reproduction is non-human and still call its products "human beings"?) Man is a maker and a selecter and a designer, and the more rationally contrived and deliberate anything is, the more human it is. Any attempt to set up an antinomy between natural and biologic reproduction, on the one hand, and artificial or designed reproduction, on the other, is absurd. The real difference is between accidental or random reproduction and rationally willed or chosen reproduction. In either case it will be biologic—according to the nature of the biologic process. If it is unnatural it can be so only in the sense that all medicine is.

It seems to me that laboratory reproduction is radically human compared to conception by ordinary heterosexual intercourse. It is willed, chosen, purposed, and controlled, and surely these are among the traits that distinguish *Homo sapiens* from others in the animal genus, from the primates down. Coital reproduction is, therefore, less human than laboratory reproduction—more fun, to be sure, but with our separation of baby making from lovemaking, both become more human because they are matters of choice, and not chance. This is, of course, essentially the case for planned parenthood. I cannot see how either humanity or morality are served by genetic roulette sexually.

The fact is that most of our discourse about the ethics of biomedical innovation is a semantic jungle, because what we mean by "human" and *ergo* by "humanistic" usually remains vague and poorly defined. The question, What is it to be human? is, however, no longer just an academic exercise for philosophers. Physicians and nurses, as well as geneticists and laboratory technicians, face it every day thousands of times. For them it is literally a life-and-death practical question. It arises *in utero* or *in vitro* when sacrifices are indicated, and it arises *in terminus* when decisions have to be made whether to go on prolonging a patient's dying. When does a fetus become human (the better term is "personal")? when is a dying patient no longer so?

Let me suggest a conceptual approach that might be adopted. In the light of medical proposals to redefine death in terms of irreversible coma or a loss of the higher brain function ("cerebral") (it might be due to a massive hemorrhage, or a neoplasm, or a trauma), if such an excerebral or decorticate patient is no longer alive in any human sense or personal sense, would it not follow that a pre-cerebral embryo or fetus is not yet alive in any human and personal sense? This would, of course, obviate any further use of such question-begging rhetoric as "killing unborn babies."

In any case, what is called for here, for consequentialists, is a quality-of-life ethics instead of the sanctity-of-life ethics in the classical Western tradition. The metarational premise or *a priori* that mere life or biologic process is sacrosanct is not only neither verifiable nor falsifiable; by logical inference it is inconsistent with empirical and humanistic medicine, as well as opposed to genetic and embryologic investigation.

The uncomfortable truth is that we have not yet put our heads together in an interdisciplinary way to see if we can find some "common-ground" factors and operational terms for such synthetic concepts as 'human' and 'personal.' Some moralists—for example, Gustafson—doubt if a consensus on 'humanness' is possible, but it is worth a try. This may well be the most searching and fundamental problem that faces not only ethicists but society as a whole.

It is already very late. It is urgent that scientists, philosophers, sociologists, lawyers, and theologians make the attempt, especially if nondoctrinaire auspices can be found. What makes a creature human? A certain level of cerebrocortical function? Self-awareness and self-control? Memory? A sense of futurity, of time? A capacity for interpersonal relationship? Communication? Love? A certain measurable I.Q.? Could we add a desire to live? What else? And in what order would we rank them as priorities?

Surely Senator Mondale was on the right track when he tried as early as 1968 to persuade Congress to propose a National Commission on Health, Science and Society. It was obstructed by people in research medicine objecting to any outside "interference." The alternative to such a thoughtful review of the implications of biomedical pioneering is apt to be hasty, unconsidered legislation. There is, indeed, a palpable danger of a new Luddism, biologic this time instead of industrial. Little as we should like to be manipulated by what Gerald Leach has called "the biocrats," neither do we want to be paralyzed by know-nothingism.

Science deals with the possible and the probable, but ethics deals with the preferable—and it is to this level of analysis that the issue of designed genetic changes in man has at last brought us. We cannot any longer sweep it under the rug.

My second point has to do with what we mean by rights. Reactionaries cannot, of course, "prove" that reproduction is ethical only when it is done heterosexually within the monogamous marriage bond, or that any one set of values or any one preferential order is the correct one, or that particular rights alleged by this group or that are sacrosanct. None of them is. For example, we cannot establish a supposed right to be born— to say nothing of what one theologian has called a "right to be born with a unique genotype."[13] (By this, of course, he can only mean the accidental genotype resulting from random or so-called natural conception, and even so, identical twins can and do occur in nature.) All alleged rights are at best imperfect and relative. But what is there, then, to appeal to, to validate our humanistic concerns and our person-centered values?

My answer is: needs. Needs are the moral stabilizers, not rights. The legalistic temper gives first place to rights, but the humanistic temper puts needs in the driver's seat. If human rights conflict with human needs, let needs prevail. If medical care can use genetic controls preventively to protect people from disease or deformity, or to ameliorate such things, then let the so-called right to be born step aside. If research with embryos and fetal tissue is needed to give us the means to cure and prevent the tragedies of "unique genotypes," even though it involves the sacrifice of some conceptuses, then let rights take a back seat.

Rights are nothing but a formal recognition by society of certain human needs, and as needs change with changing conditions, so rights should change, too. The right to conceive and bear children has to stop short of knowingly making crippled children—and genetics gives us that knowledge—just as the rights of parents have had to bow to required schooling, and the rights of voluntary association have had to bow, in public services, to the human need to be respected regardless of ethnic and racial differences. It is human need that validates rights, not the other way around. I for one am not primarily concerned about any claimed rights to live or to die; I am first of all concerned about human needs, and whether they are met by life or by death will depend on the situation.

To speak of needs is to speak of human values. How shall we identify and rank-order them? Here, again, we have to have across-the-board cultural consultation. I agree with Michael Baram, of MIT, who says:

> I do not think scientific peer groups presently have the objectivity or capability to function as coherent and humane social controls. The members of a peer group share the narrow confines of their discipline, and individual success is measured by the degree to which one plunges more deeply into and more narrowly draws the bounds of his research. There are no peer group rewards for activities or perceptions that extend beyond the discipline or relate it to social problems. Members are therefore neither motivated nor trained to relate their peer group activity to broader social problems.
>
> Self-enclosed peer groups cannot be entrusted with self-control...because our educational system does not foster ethical and interdisciplinary values in professional training.[14]

Owing to the work of microbiologists and embryologists, we are already able to produce babies born from parents who are separated by space or even by death; women are already able to nourish and gestate other women's children; one man can "father" thousands of children; virgin births or parthenogenesis, as well as cloning, are likely soon to be feasible; by genetic intervention we can shape babies, rather than doing so only from the seed of our loins; artificial wombs and placentas are projected by biochemists and pharmacologists. All this means that we are going to have to change or alter our old ideas about who or what a father is, or a mother, or a family. Francis Crick, co-describer of DNA, and others are quite right to say that all this is going to destroy to some extent our traditional grounds for ethical beliefs.

But whatsoever new mental images take shape within new situations, as long as they are tailored to a loving concern for human beings, we need not be afraid. Fear is at the bottom of this debate—some of it the conventional wisdom's fear of change, some of it a fear of science, and some of it fear of freedom's power and creative control. It is, perhaps, the fear of fear itself that makes for a lot of blocks and evasions. But however that may be, the historic moral order has always presupposed heterosexual coital conception as necessary for the continuance of life, and now that is no longer the case. The familiar phrase "the facts of life" is an archaism.

I agree with Roger Shinn that in the sequence or progression from aspirin to insulin to artificial kidneys to brain surgery to genetic engineering there is no point at which we can "change from a clear yes to an absolute no," even though there is a mounting difference in the complexity of the ethical issues posed.[15] We cannot accept the "invisible hand" of blind natural chance or random nature in genetics any more than we could Professor Jevon's theory of feast and famine in nineteenth-century laissez-faire economics based on sun spots and tidal movements. To be men we must be in control. That is the first and last ethical word. For when there is no choice, there is no possibility of ethical action. Whatever we are compelled to do is amoral.

The moral philosopher, sensitive to social ethics, can only echo what biologist Robert Sinsheimer has said: "As the discoveries accumulate, as new means of biological intervention arise, we can envision such possibilities as the almost indefinite prolongation of life for at least a few, the deliberate predetermination of sex, or the design of human genetic change for varied purposes. With these will come the necessity for multiple social decisions of the most profound consequence."[16]

The pressure of social decision making is now forcing us to dig deeper than the technical hardware sciences; we now have to grapple with the personal and human software sciences—especially biology and the crossroads it reveals to us, just ahead.

1. Britannica *Book of the Year 1964* (Chicago: Encyclopedia Britannica, Inc., 1964), 499-500.

2. A. Rosenfeld, *The Second Genesis: The Coming Control of Life* (Englewood Cliffs, New Jersey: Prentice-Hall, 1969), 145.

3. Michael Hamilton, "New Life for Old: Genetic Decisions," *Christian Century* 86 (1969), 741-744.

4. Richard McCormick, "Notes on Moral Theology," *Theological Studies* 30 (1969), 680-692.

5. J.B.S. Haldane, "Biological Possibilities for the Human Species in the Next Ten Thousand Years," in *Man and His Future*, ed. G. Wolstenholme (Boston: Little, Brown and Company, 1963), 337-361.

6. Theodosius Dobzhansky, *Heredity and the Nature of Man* (New York: Harcourt, Brace and World, 1964).

7. Leon Kass, "New Beginnings in Life," in *The New Genetics and the Future of Man* ed. M. Hamilton (Grand Rapids, Michigan: Eerdmans Publishing Company, 1972), 30.

8. Paul Ramsey, "Moral and Religious Implications of Genetic Control," in *Genetics and the Future of Man*, ed J. D. Roslansky (Amsterdam: North-Holland Publishing Company, 1966), 107-169.

9. James Gustafson, "Basic Ethical Issues in the Biomedical Fields", *Soundings* 52 (1970), 151-180.

10. Jeremy Bentham, "The Influence of Time and Place in Matters of Legislation," in *The Works of Jeremy Bentham*, ed. J. Bowring vol. 1. (London: Simpkin, Marshall, and Company, 1843), 169-194.

11. Joshua Lederberg, "Genetic Engineering, or the Amelioration of Genetic Defect," *Pharos* 34 (1971), 9-12.

12. André Helleger, Letter to the editor, *Washington Post*, January 9, 1971, A21.

13. Paul Ramsey, *Fabricated Man: The Ethics of Genetic Control* (New Haven: Yale University Press, 1970).

14. Michael S. Baram, "Social Control of Science and Technology," *Science* 172 (1971), 535-539.

15. Roger Shinn, "The Ethics of Genetic Engineering" *North Dakota State University Bulletin*, April 22, 1967, 13-21.

16. Robert Sinsheimer, "The Implications of Recent Advances in Biology for the Future of Medicine," *Engineering Science* 34 (1970), 6-13.

Eight

Fetal Research

We want our people, especially our children, to be safe from disease of any kind, including genetic and congenital disorders, uterine infections, and a host of other birth maladies. This means we have to learn as much as we can about controlling reproduction, to be free as much as possible from the dangers of blind, natural cause-and-effect. Individual scientists, of course, may be moved by an intellectual itch and/or a hunger for fame, but the main thing is human well-being.

How can we continue to achieve vital research benefits for reproductive medicine, while maintaining at the same time a high ethical standard of concern for human subjects? In this appraisal of the problem I will contend that fetuses are not human beings except in the purely biological sense of the phrase, even though they are *potentially* persons. What, then, do we owe them?

Virtually all that is known of some branches of reproductive medicine has come from clinical research; techniques for antenatal diagnosis, for example, have been acquired through fetal research *in utero*. The Nuremberg code is definite: clinical experimentation, i.e. experiments using human subjects, usually patients, is justified if it can be hoped it will yield "fruitful results...unprocurable by other methods and means."

One survey of attitudes has reported that clinical researchers do not rate ethical concern very high. It asked the question, "What characteristics do you want to know about another researcher before entering into a collaborative relationship...?" The response was 86% "scientific ability," 45% "hard work," 43% "personality," and only 6% "ethical concern for research subjects."[1] However, it should be noted that the respondents were first of all concerned for competence; that, after all, is their first ethical obligation to their subjects. The mere fact that "concern for research subjects" did not leap to mind is certainly not an indication they care nothing about their subjects, as any very wide acquaintance with physicians will show.

People often think that ethics means finding something that is "bad," *as such*, and then categorically forbidding it by a rule of morality. This is, alas, one kind of ethics. However, in this appraisal, as John Dewey would have called it, a hypothetical rather than a categorical ethics will be employed. In this kind of ethics the moral agent says, "This or that is not wrong if it leads foreseeably to consequences deemed to be desirable." Rightness and wrongness are judged according to results, not according to absolute prohibitions or demands. The ethics here, then, is not categorical, based on prescriptive norms; it is not ideological nor rule-determined. On the contrary, it is based on the principle of proportionate good; it is consequential, pragmatic, and value-determined.

To illustrate the point, neither amniocentesis nor fetoscopy is as yet entirely without risk as a diagnostic procedure. There is some risk in the aspiration of amniotic fluid and in the use of cannulas and lenses to examine fetuses suspected of being aberrant or diseased, for example, in getting blood samples in a suspected hemoglobin disorder like betathalassemia. The procedure is still experimental, however slightly; it is still investigative medicine. One state's law actually bans it as a nonbeneficial risk to a live fetus. Yet three out of four times such a diagnosis would yield "all is well" or "signs negative"—a preponderantly good consequence. In this perspective, therefore, it is held to be a good thing because it eliminates the risk of terminating healthy pregnancies out of fear of getting a defective baby.

The state law just mentioned was passed on the ground that *all* nonbeneficial risks to a fetus are wrong as such, regardless of whether we could weigh up the benefits and discover that in some cases they more than make up for whatever the risks and costs might be. The fact that it would save many babies is not, in doctrinaire ethics, allowed to weigh against the categorical condemnation. Its followers would say, "*All* experimental risks to live fetuses are *ipso facto* unethical, no matter how good the consequences." (One religious moralist has even argued, in addition, that it is unethical because the fetus has not given its consent nor ever could—rather like those who condemn abortion, regardless of any good consequences to be gained.)

Pappworth puts it very bluntly. "Whether an experiment [has] gained its desired result or not is to me immaterial... A worthy end does not justify unworthy means... Every human being has the right to be treated with decency and that right belongs to each and every individual and should supersede every consideration of what *may* advance medical science. No doctor is justified in placing science or the public welfare first and his obligation to his patient second."[2] Here we have a whole battery of ethical assertions, all of which will have to be rejected or seriously qualified: his radical individualism, the notion that the end cannot ever justify the means, an appeal to "rights" as if they were perfect and unconditional, and an undisclosed but obviously quite subjective understanding of "decency."

This brief discussion of ethical alternatives shows how a pragmatic ethics based on values, quality of life, and proportionate good differs from a dogmatic ethics of rules and categorical judgments and prejudicial (prejudiced) decision making. It also helps the reader to know what ethical rules of the game are being followed here. Now let us turn to the question itself, as analyzed by an ethicist who is neither a biologist nor a physician.

The core question at stake in the ethics of fetal research is whether a fetus is a person. Very soon after fertilization it is apparent that the conceptus or embryo is biologically of the human species, and that it is living in the sense that cell division is going on furiously. But are we to assign personal status to a fetus, i.e., render it the regard and rights we grant to living, breathing, independently functioning individuals?

The contention that we should assign human rights to the fetus is a familiar one, yet one definitely rejected by the Supreme Court. In *Roe* v. *Wade* (1973) this question was decided in terms which uphold the ethics of relative values—namely, that fetuses are not persons, although any state may (but not must) choose to protect fetal life from termination in some cases in the third trimester, but not until then and only if it finds it has a "compelling interest" in the *potential* (postnatal) person. The Court itself, then, did not proscribe even third trimester abortions in such procedures as hysterotomies and saline induction—prior to viability. The logic of the decision is to validate not only terminating pregnancies by the induced abortion of previable fetuses, but the forestalling of unwanted live births late in pregnancy—undesirable as it might be medically in most such cases.

An actual person, as distinguished from a potential one, is therefore both legally and ethically a human being who has left the maternal-fetal unit, is born alive, and lives entirely outside the mother's body with an independent cardiovascular system. Only the pregnant patient is a "human subject" to be protected in clinical experimentation and research; the fetus is an object, not a subject—a nonpersonal organism.

A fetus is "precious" or "has value" only when its potentiality is *wanted*. This means when it is wanted by the progenitors, not by somebody else. Hence the principle of privacy, of control of one's own body and its product, except that some states *might* intervene to do the wanting after twenty-four weeks of gestation. The courts have held further that if a fetus is wanted by one progenitor but not the other, then the mother has the initiative, either to carry it to term or to abort.

The metaphysical or religious belief that fetuses are persons is a perfectly legitimate act of faith, but there is no way to prove it or show it; by reason of its nonempirical nature as a faith assertion it cannot be either verified or falsified. Most of us, when we look at the consequences of that belief, reject it because consistently acting on it would lower the quality of life in our children and paralyze our standards of reproductive medicine. To treat live fetuses as untouchable is absurd. Variables such as their functional condition and health prospects, costs of treatment both financially and emotionally, maternal consent, the need to "touch" them by medical interventions, whether they are destined for termination—these factors should enter into the decisional mix.

The fetus is not a patient. A patient is a person. The Hippocratic Oath does not recognize the fetus as a person—unless you want to infer it from the archaic statement, "I will not give to a woman a pessary to produce an abortion." The World Medical Association's reduction of the Oath leaves it out altogether, declaring only that the "utmost respect for human life from the time of its conception" should be maintained, leaving open what "respect" and "conception" are to mean.

Dr. Joshua Lederberg sees the problem in a nondoctrinaire way, as do the great majority. Speaking of governmental proposals to limit fetus research, he said, "The crux of the matter is whether one views the abortus [sic] as a person..."[3] He was replying to Dr. Andre Hellegers, a doctrinaire moralist of the minority, whose contention was that "no one can give consent to an experiment on [a live] aborted fetus... It would be like asking consent from a parent who had abandoned or battered a child."[4]

Here we have a moral disagreement in good faith. One side thinks vitalistically, that where there is fetal life it is sacrosanct; the other side determines the issue by quality of life considerations. One side looks at persons as events or endowments (e.g., "infusion of the soul"), while the other sees persons as a process or an achievement developmentally. This is obviously not a matter to be decided by government fiat. The First

Amendment to the Constitution forbids any such solution in a pluralist democracy. In short, there should be no compulsory pregnancy or motherhood, and by the same token no compulsory abortion or fetal research.

The ethics of fetal research has had remarkably little discussion. For example, in the 1154 pages of Jay Katz's compendium on the ethics and law of human experimentation, *Experimentation with Human Beings*, there are *fewer than a half dozen* pages given to fetal research. What we are to think about probing fetal life *in utero* and *ex utero*, in order to prolong the life of children yet to be born or of children already born, is still very much open to exploration and certainly open to differences of opinion and practice. Physicians and scientists will have to decide pretty largely for themselves whether to learn how to save living human beings by the use of whole fetuses, fetal tissues, or fetal materials. Each investigator, for example, will have to decide for himself or herself whether—to take a couple of examples—to perfuse abortuses to develop ways to prevent spontaneous abortions, or to prevent drug toxicity in fetuses going to term. All should be free to participate or not to participate.

Expressed in philosophical language, as I have remarked, the question is whether a fetus is an object or a subject. If, as we suppose here, the fetus is not a subject, then it follows that "protection of human subjects" in fetal research can only mean protection of pregnant women and live-born babies, pre-term and full-term, not of previable fetuses *in utero* or *ex utero*.

A related issue is whether persons or subjects have to be actual or only potential to be real human beings. What is called in logic the 'error of potentiality' is to confuse what is yet to be or could be, with what is. It supposes that because a fetus could possibly or probably become a person, it is therefore a person *now*. Viability anticipated converts somehow into viability realized. This 'prolepsis' falsifies reality; in its eagerness it slips into thinking that what we want is already possessed, when in fact we are only hoping for it. In fact, a fetus is precisely and only a fetus.[5]

There seems to be good reason to question both the validity and usefulness of the concept of viability, at least as a stage of gestation having any ethical significance. Modern resuscitation and artificial life-support technologies are pushing "viability" farther and farther back towards nidation—possibly to four weeks. Marginal errors about gestational age are inevitable, in spite of such devices as ultrasound measurements of fetal head diameter. At present, infants of seven hundred grams are probably the baseline, even though efforts are made to save those of six hundred grams if parents want it done. Yet research and development on synthetic placentas and artificial uteruses is extending the incubation period we now have for premature infants, prematurity representing the greatest mortality frequency in perinatal medicine. The date of viability is sure to be pushed back, until at last its relevance to speculations about humanness and personhood will have become absurd. Those who are hung up on the resemblance of the fetal morphon to a live-born baby will be released progressively from that psychological trap, called the "homunculus reaction."

Such notions are always changing, as medicine's capabilities change. Viability used to mean a fetus was capable of spontaneous functioning at separation from the mother. Then it came to mean (for some, not all) being capable of functioning by artificial means until spontaneous functioning begins. Soon it will come to mean being kept going artificially at any stage *beginning with fertilization*. Arguments about *"prima facie* viability" at twenty-eight weeks or twenty-four weeks or twenty weeks are superficial and increasingly irrelevant to the question of survivability of fetal life. One government official has said, "If you have a viable fetus you are in precisely the same position as you would be with a minor child," but thought-forms like that more and more take on the appearance of the grotesque. Throughout the centuries the term viability has meant, literally, "ability to live"—to live apart from maternal-placental support. No artificial support was available. But now, with respirators and the new biochemistry of lung inflation, who is to say what the word will come to mean, as to either the fetus's development or its ectogenetic independence of the human uterus?

Guidelines laid down in the past by the National Institutes of Health try to avoid the pitfalls of viability's definition. They have made it a matter of simple heartbeat and respiration, and thus required that no "harm" be done to fetuses *regardless* of head size, gram weight, physiological development, genetic diseases, congenital anomalies. Viability obtains just whenever and simply because the fetal heart beats and because it breathes. This disregard of quality-of-life factors is very upsetting; it is unacceptably undiscriminating and inhumane. The question is not whether a fetus has vital signs, but whether it should be brought to live birth. If not, then surely research and experimentation are in order. A Tay-Sachs fetus *in utero* is alive; so is a massively lesioned myelomeningocele prematurely expelled, *ex utero*. With proper consent, learning from such false starts should be allowed as entirely ethical.

In America's pluralist society variety and differences of belief and values are essential. They provide the creative abrasion of competition and inquiry. Such disagreements, ethical as well as religious and cultural, are just as vital to the progress of reproductive medicine as they are to all other human enterprises. Homogenization of opinion would be a disaster to science as well as to medical care and treatment if any particular set of pre- or metaethical assumptions about personhood and humanhood in fetal life were to be given a monopoly force by law, or by funding work which must be done exclusively according to only one system of ethics and rules for obstetrics, gynecology, perinatology, and pediatrics.

Quite apart from its being wrong to impose such rules, they would surely be evaded and violated, thereby encouraging the dishonesty which always grows up under a Big Brother and authoritarian policy. Many people's belief propositions are entirely visceral, not rational—witness, for example, the repugnance some people feel at perfusion of a separated fetus head while feeling none at the perfusion of its kidney. Where we start from is essentially important in understanding our own moral judgments, and others', but to force us all into the same value mold would be a moralistic dictatorship.

Our most searching ethical question has to do with live fetus research, not the use of abortuses and fetal tissues and materials. After vital signs are gone, fetuses are in the domain of autopsy and pathological examination. The issue was drawn by temporary regulations of the Department of Health, Education and Welfare banning all nontherapeutic live fetus research *in utero*, whether the fetus is viable or previable, and even if the fetus is destined for abortion and the research has the patient's consent. The regulations banned the use of artificial life support for research purposes, even when a fetus is determined to be not viable, because it would be (obviously) nontherapeutic and not intended to "save" the life of the fetus.

Here we have an instance of a dogmatic or doctrinaire condemnation of something as intrinsically wrong, regardless of any extrinsic consideration of the benefits to be gained. Common sense, in any case, does not allow that a fetus which is inviable or to be terminated can be "harmed" or "injured" or "insulted," since acts of battery and mayhem presuppose a living, independent individual. Invasive treatment of a fetus, in either therapy or experimentation, might come under the heading in law of mutilation, as of a corpse, but would not be an injury (*iniure*, or "injustice"). An injustice predicates a person. The only injury could be to the maternal patient, and with the appropriate consent even that becomes null.

In a way, NIH was putting itself in the position of assigning rights to a fetus *in utero*. If, as this appraisal maintains, a fetus is without personal status, the ban in effect assigned human rights to a nonperson, which is precisely what the Supreme Court has set aside. It is a repudiation of the judiciary by an agency of the executive. Its effect is to reduce our knowledge of fetal physiology and medicine to anecdotal observation instead of the genuine research which is vital to completely verified and reliable life-saving information.

As a part of this temporary policy, a ban was also laid on keeping fetuses going *ex utero* by artificial supports for a few hours (seven or eight at the most), even though the fetus is not ultimately viable—in the original sense of being or becoming able to function independently of the maternal womb. In the same mood in which they banned the use of artificial support systems to keep fetal life going for research purposes, artificial systems to get life *started* were also banned—as in the case of *in vitro* fertilization and implantation. (The 1972 "Peel report" of an advisory group on fetal research in Great Britain also asserted, in a somewhat sweeping fashion, that it is "unethical" to do any fetal research *in utero* aimed at "ascertaining the harm" drugs and procedures might do. Their ban did not extend to studies of fetuses *ex utero*, however; they allowed use of such fetuses as, simply, "previables." Their opposition, by the way, was not based on any assertion of fetal rights but on the danger to experimenters of law suits by disappointed or disgruntled patients.)[6]

But what is of the most urgent importance is that the NIH rules did not disclose *any explanation at all of the prohibitions, nor of the assertion that such research is unethical.* In a civilized, democratic society it is unthinkable that regulations and prohibitions may be laid upon scientists and healers in fiat form, *without any disclosure or defense of the reasons* for them. Ethically speaking, this is a point of critical significance. Rules without a rationale cut straight across the principle of "due process" and are, as lawyers like to say, "arbitrary and capricious."

The tension between life-saving research and prohibitions of fetal research is very real. There is a considerable body of information needed, which is to be gained only from experiments and investigations with live fetuses *in* or *ex utero*; abortus research does not meet the need. We have to know more about detecting diseases in pregnant mothers, reducing the hazards of induced abortion, identifying which donor-fetal tissue—thymus, liver, spleen, and so on—will save deficient newborns (for example, agammaglobulinaemia children), and we need to study abnormalities.

It has been argued (consequentially) that fetal research would have a brutalizing effect on us all if it were to be countenanced, but surely the reply is that it *has* been done without that effect, before it was brought to a halt. A more brutalizing effect would follow if we should refuse to learn how to avert fetal disorders and how to avoid bringing disordered babies into the world, *knowing that we could prevent such misery.* Live fetus research can help to prevent the twenty to thirty percent of wanted pregnancies lost in spontaneous abortion. Experiments with maternal-fetal patients whose pregnancies are to be aborted can achieve impressive gains for life and health, for example, tests of rubella vaccine by injecting the mothers, and tests of drugs to determine what substances a fetus can absorb or which ones can cross the placental barrier.

Fetal experiments should be done *ex utero* to develop incubator procedures for prolonging the life of possibly viable premature fetuses, to carry them along until they can survive and enter the nursery; to find treatments for asphyxiated newborns (e.g., complete perfusion); to test artificial placentas to help a newborn with respiratory distress syndrome; to learn about fetal physiology; to fight birth defects, diagnose disorders, and reduce neonatal mortality and morbidity.

Furthermore, research with nonviable live fetuses could lead the way to therapeutic gains such as the use of thymus for "Swiss type" agammaglobulinaemia, donor transplant tissue, fetal organs for use in biochemistry, tissue cultures for vaccines, and liver-lung-and-spleen tissue for measles and polio vaccines, and to increase the accuracy of amniocentesis. The Peel report in Britain listed 51 specific *in utero* and *ex utero* experiments and research goals with live fetuses, of importance to reproduction and general medicine.

The moralistic temper which strives for ever more restrictive regulations comes from an ethical stance in which life *qua* life, regardless of its quality, is the first-order value. Many of us, on the other hand, opt for quality, not quantity, with the value judgment that sometimes life is not worth living. Only if we are "sacralists," investing life with a sacred entelechy of some kind, would we want to put a taboo on direct human control over life.

We see this issue underneath both the fetal research debate and the terminal care debate. The issue runs through nearly all biomedical policy—transplants, determination of death, triage, and many other problems. Quality or value ethics requires us to transvaluate our values; we cannot dogmatically put being alive as the highest good. Life is a value to be perceived in relation to other values. At best it is only *primus inter pares.* Without life, of course, nothing else is of any value to us, but, by the same token, without some other things life may be of no value either.

A curious aspect of the consent problem is that *compulsory motherhood* is the result if there is a requirement to save all viable fetuses. For example, if a women's elective abortion came very late and the fetus was by rule artificially supported up to viability, it would mean making her a mother against her will. In such rules the consent of patients to live fetus research, *in utero* and *ex utero*, is nullified in spite of her choice and her physician's.

Dr. Robert Goodlin's work at Stanford on live previable fetuses, including the product of hysterotomies (one fetus was kept alive for eleven days) was as successful as it was because so many patients asked him to do their terminations, wanting some good to come of their unpleasant experience. The NIH prohibitions, unreasoned and unexplained, nullified all such compassionate efforts to help save fetuses born with immature and uninflatable lungs.[7] This was a serious invasion of free consent, and especially serious since it is a policy imposed by those who otherwise make a great parade of respect for the patient's consent as something which should always be sought.

One of the lurking ethical issues in fetal research is the means-ends controversy. Is risking damage to fetal life always wrong, an intrinsically evil act? A categorical moralist might see it that way. Presumably, if fetal life is personal it would be looked on as mayhem, battery, or even felonious assault. But looked at hypothetically and pragmatically, whether intended or unintended, damage to a fetus is wrong would depend upon such variables as whether it was to be terminated anyway, and whether the good to be gained would outweigh the damage suffered. In a nondoctrinaire ethics, proportionate good or a favorable cost-benefit ratio would decide it. (For those who do not believe a fetus is a person there is no question of "murder" or "manslaughter" or "unlawful death" in abortion or fetal research, but only of choosing to lose or forego a potential person.)

As Franz Ingelfinger, the editor of *The New England Journal of Medicine*, once expressed it, to be right "the desired end should always be of sufficient value to justify the means..."[8] In every profession serving human needs the good and bad have to be weighed relatively. Ethical analysis is choosing between alternatives. The moral agent is a chooser in the clinical or case-focused spirit, not a straight-down-the-line follower of prefabricated decisional rules. When Dr. Pappworth, as quoted earlier, says that whether an experiment gains the desired results is "immaterial" to him, because a "worthy end does not justify unworthy means," we have to part company; his categorical rigidity is ethically irresponsible.

The objection to letting people be free moral agents, to judge what is best in each situation, is never given in the doctrinaire terms which undergird it; it comes in the shape of an objection called the "slippery slope" or the "thin edge of the wedge." Where there is a trade-off between protecting fetal life and saving "born" life or learning how to do it, they complain that a "domino effect" will go into play and that if allowed such medical studies will end up in a re-enactment of the "Nazi situation" or *"Brave New World"* or *"1984."* (The Nazi atrocities perpetrated in the name of medical research were, of course, blatant and ruthless experiments carried out on involuntary and uniformed subjects.)

This parade of horrors is not logical or rational analysis ethically; it is a mood objection, not a reasoned one. There is hardly a single advance in scientific know-how which could not conceivably be turned to stupid and malicious misuses and abuses. (There is no "answer" to the objection because there is no analyzable question posed; it is not an argument to be refuted.)

The 'fallacy of necessity' lies behind the wedge objection—the notion, that is, that because we *can* do something it is certain that we *will* do it. Or, more carefully expressed, we will do it uncritically and undiscriminatingly. Prudence, an ancient and essential virtue, might sometimes turn us against an experiment or research study in fetal medicine because the gain would not be proportionate to the cost, the flame not worth the candle. That is prudence. The wedge objection, on the other hand, as in the case of live fetus research or invasive therapy, is imprudent or anti-prudent, since it rejects all responsible ethical judgment with a blanket ban, *ab initio*. It repudiates critical analysis in favor of taboo.

Our problem is political as much as ethical. How are we to live and let live in American medicine, which functions in a pluralist society composed of varying and even contradictory beliefs and values?

Shall we who are pragmatic and value-oriented compromise with the "pro-lifers" who are doctrinaire and rule-oriented, or should we both follow laissez-faire? How are we to show our concern and tolerance for minority sentiments, by compromise or by full freedom of conscience? Shall we ban some categories of live fetus research and allow others, or should we put aside "class actions" and individuate cases, allowing the minority moralists to choose for themselves in every case whether they will participate or not?

Unhappily but necessarily, if rules are imposed by law or public agencies, somebody is frustrated, one group or the other. In matters of this kind there is great wisdom in the old adage, the best government is the least government. The issue cannot be resolved satisfactorily to all. Ethically regarded, the anti-research forces might be comforted; they would not have to engage in any research that violates their consciences. (One tart suggestion is that we ought to compile a list for them of all the drugs and procedures that have been or will be derived from live fetus research, so that they can avoid using them for the protection and health of their own children. Anti-fetal research agitators are as inconsistent on this score as the antivivisectionists.)

We have reached five summary conclusions about fetal research:

1. It is justifiable, depending on the clinical situation and the design, to make any use of abortuses or dead fetuses—whole, tissues, or uterine materials—whether from voluntary or therapeutic abortions, and with or without maternal consent.

2. It is justifiable, depending on the clinical situation and the design, to make any use of live fetuses *ex utero*, previable or viable, if survival is not purposed or wanted, and if there is maternal consent.

3. It is justifiable, depending on the clinical situation and the design, to make any use of live fetuses *in utero*, if survival is not purposed or wanted, and if there is maternal consent.

4. It is justifiable, depending on the clinical situation and the design, to use live fetuses *in utero* even if survival is intended, if there is no substantial risk to the fetus, and if there is both maternal and spouse-paternal consent.

5. As a fifth finding we may add the point already discussed, that regulations by the public authority are unethical if the reasons for them, the ethics they are rested upon, are not disclosed fully and frankly.

To say that the best government is the least government does not mean that government is wholly evil, nor even that it can be called a "necessary evil." Necessary, yes, but not evil. Fetal research and experimentation should not be radically individualistic nor a laissez-faire program carried out by personal whim without any kind of monitoring and control.

Two physicians a year or so ago wrote letters to *The Journal of the American Medical Association* to protest against a paper which had favored fetal research. Their complaint was that the writers of the paper had sold out to "an ethic of expedience"—which they rejected because it "favors utility above principle."[9] Apparently without realizing it, they put their fingers precisely on the main issue: categorical rules versus weighing pros and cons. If "principles" block medicine's healing task, so much the worse for principles. We must be delivered from the kind of ethics which follows principles when following them means we have to condemn and nullify the acquisition of useful know-how in medicine's effort to save and improve human life.

1. B. Barber, et al., "Experimenting with Humans: Problems and Process of Social Control in the Biomedical Research Community," in *The Challenge of Life*: *Bio-medical* |

Progress and Human Values (Roche Anniversary Symposium) (Basel and Stuttgart: Birkhauer Verlag, 1972), 357-370.

2. M. H. Pappworth, M.D., "Ethical Issues in Experimental Medicine," in *Updating Life and Death*, (Boston: Beacon Press, 1969), 64-84.

3. *World Medical News*, October 5, 1973, p. 36.

4. Ibid.

5. Joseph Fletcher, *The Ethics of Genetic Control* (New York: Doubleday/Anchor, 1974), 91, 137-139.

6. "The Use of Fetuses and Fetal Material for Research," Department of Health and Social Security, (London: Her Majesty's Stationery Office, 1972), 6.

7. *World Medical News*, October 5, 1973, p. 33.

8. *The New England Journal of Medicine* 269 (1962) 479. He was discussing experiments on children, but his reasoning fitted fetal experiments too.

9. Franz Ingelfinger, *Journal of the American Medical Association* 230 (1974) 1124.

Nine

Our Duty to the Unborn

"Sexually Transmissible Disease" is the title of an article in the World Health Organization's monthly magazine *World Health* for May, 1975. The article contains not a single word about genetic diseases: only venereal diseases are mentioned. This perspective has been entirely outmoded by scientific and clinical human genetics. The range of modern preventive medicine is far too wide for that kind of tunnel vision.

The concept of communicable disease is now radically revised by our having learned how diseases are vertically communicated, from one generation to another, as well as horizontally communicated from one contemporary to another. Inescapably the question arises, If infectious diseases are in some cases serious enough to justify public or legal control of their transmission, why not genetic diseases too? What is our intergenerational responsibility?

Prevention and treatment of genetic diseases, as of infectious diseases, is quite feasible—increasingly so. The only difference is that one kind spreads by contagion and the other by reproduction. The question posed by medical genetics is ethical: not *can* genetic disorders be controlled, but *ought* they. Involved are medical problems still unsolved and legal problems still unresolved, but the basic issue is an ethical one. At bottom it seems to be this: Should society use law both to treat and to prevent genetic disorders? (Presumably only some genetic disorders, not all.)

Ethics and law are closer to each other than to medicine and its foundation in biology. Sciences as such are descriptive, knowledge-oriented, concerned with what is, whereas law and ethics (moral philosophy) are prescriptive, value-oriented, and concerned with what ought to be. Both ethics and law, therefore, attempt as convincingly as possible to recommend policies and courses of action. Justice and rightness are only peripheral in science, but the very substance of ethics and law. There is plenty of evidence, as we shall be seeing, that bioethics finds its most suggestive and crucial clues in the interface between law and ethics. That interface is jurisprudence, in the meaning lexicographers give it as their first definition: the philosophy of law.

Law and ethics are alerted most fully, and their critical concern is most fully aroused, whenever a policy or practice is imposed by involuntary or compulsory means. In what follows we will be taking a close look at just such a proposal, and we will find that Justice Frankfurter's reference to the "legal thicket" has its parallel in the ethical thicket.[1]

THE ISSUE

Let us compare two situations. First, a school system specialist in judo instruction unknowingly carries meningococcus bacteria, although, like the storied Typhoid Mary, he is himself uninfected.[2] Several high school students fall ill, and the public health authorities finally trace it to the instructor. When he chooses not to accept treatment, he is placed in detention, then forced to accept treatment. His rights of privacy, movement, employment of his own choosing, personal bodily integrity, and consent—all are denied. It was a temporary but not permanent restraint.

In the second situation, a housewife unknowingly carries the autosomal dominant gene for Huntington's chorea. When she tells her physician of recent paranoidal personality changes in her two sisters, a genetic diagnosis reveals that she and her sisters are at fifty percent risk of the disease. The patient refuses to be sterilized—which would be a permanent and not merely temporary restraint. Is not such a "quarantine" in order here too? (If the offspring of all affecteds were sterilized, Huntington's chorea would be wiped out in one generation's time.) The two diseases are passed on in different ways, but both are neurological disasters for others—most of all for the innocent victims conceived and born by the carriers.

We are concerned here primarily with a problem in medicine, not in social biology or genetic engineering. The reigning view in our society, among those who have given the question any serious examination, is that voluntary controls of genetic disorders, by free parental choice, is the ideal way to deal with the problem. "Ideal" in this context sometimes means "most effective" and other times "morally best." We shall find there are reasons to doubt that voluntary controls are always ideal, in either sense.

In situations of genetic disorder, four parties of interest are involved. There are not only (1) the parents or prospective parents, but (2) the potential children, involving also (3) the siblings and other members of the family, and more widely (4) the public or society.

Legal problems aside, and looked at only on ethical grounds, the problem comes down to three controversial issues: (1) Is it right to judge that sometimes the condition of a newborn falls below, or would fall below, a reasonable standard of quality? In short, may we set a quality standard for our progeny? (2) Are we morally obliged to avoid having children with serious genetic disorders, if and when we *can* avoid it? (3) Can we justify (ethically validate) interference by society through law to uphold minimum standards and prevent predictable misbegottens?

To reach an affirmative conclusion on the first question does not logically entail affirmative answers to either the second or third, and there are those who would contend that affirmative answers to both the first and second questions should lead to personally accepted but not legally established standards. As others see it, the first question (whether to accept quality standards in principle) is the most searching question, and to accept the principle is tantamount to accepting a law to reinforce it.

These three questions are at the heart of our problem: each of them is sure to evoke a mixed reception in popular debate. On the issue of reproductive standards, some people contend that we all recognize the right to control our own lives and our family's and that this properly includes deciding what standard of quality is best for our own children. On the other hand, some assert that every fetus has a right to be born; that out of respect for human life every conceptus should be preserved, without fear or favor. Some extremists even assert that conception should not be selectively controlled, even voluntarily, and that contraception, sterilization, and abortion are morally wrong. Still others insist that nobody is in a position to say what "normal" is in reproductive quality, and that therefore parents should be free to decide how much disease or defect in a child will hurt the family.

Some say that every child has a right to be born with a sound mind and body and we should therefore avoid knowingly depriving a child of that birthright or hurting the family and the community with the burden entailed. In this school of thought, which has judicial support, it is contended that children are not their parents' chattels and that both society in general and children in particular are better served by community standards than by the unlimited discretion of parents.

Those who oppose control argue several counter-contentions. One is that we cannot accurately foresee and measure what the burden will be, that the factors of gain-loss are not quantifiable: "dollars are dollars but feelings are feelings." In the same vein they argue that parents have no idea how much misfortune they can endure, when push comes to shove. It is also contended that the alleged right to be born sound is unrealistic and vague, not a workable concept legally or ethically. Another common point is that it is not fair to restrict carriers of genetic faults, nor restrain them, since they are not to blame for what their genes are—the assumption being that evils which are not blameworthy (imputable) ought not to be contained. Still another objection is that to outlaw defective reproduction cuts across the parents' right of free choice and self-determination (which it certainly does). It is further argued that, if there is a quality standard, those children who barely qualify will be degraded and stigmatized. A question is also raised as to *who* would set such quality standards apparently in the belief that there is no acceptable answer.

For some the third question is the thorniest, even when they agree that quality is desirable. Can we justify social intrusion because of an alleged social interest, or should quality control be entirely voluntary? Is there a substantial or "compelling" pubic interest at stake, sufficient to justify legal reinforcement of quality control? Those who think so believe that society has a vital interest in the basic genetic potential of its members-to-be, that parents should be concerned to protect that interest voluntarily, and that society through democratic law may rightly set limits on the individual's reproductive choices. This policy implies, of course, that when the private persons's sense of duty fails, society has a duty to provide a social minimum in order to contain the consequences of private failure. Such standards would have to avoid being (as lawyers might express it) capricious, arbitrary, and overbroad. Their opponents argue that ideas of social worth are hazy and debatable, that society should help parents with support funds and ameliorative care to bear the burden of misfits, that making babies is a right and not a privilege. Some even go so far as to argue that genetic disease and defects are vitally needed in order to maintain diversity in the general gene pool.[3]

There are, in addition, three anticontrol arguments of a more generalized kind. One of them tries to identify control, especially selective abortion, with Nazi attitudes as revealed in the war crimes trials after World War II. This is guilt by association, or what logicians call the fallacy of the undistributed middle. "The Nazis wanted genetic selection, those who favor control want genetic selection, *ergo* those who favor control are Nazis." (It runs into the further difficulty that, unlike the democracies, the Nazis enacted the only European law code ever to actually treat abortion as murder and punish it by death.)³ Fear that exercising human controls over reproduction will end sooner or later in elitist discrimination against "ordinary" offspring is another such objection, brought against both private and public control. This is called the slippery slope objection, to be scrutinized a bit later on. Finally, there are those who directly or indirectly reveal a basic or primary sentiment of dislike and even fear of government. They feel that the best government is the least government, holding a social philosophy of radical *laissez faire*. Hence they oppose *public* control, even though they might favor *voluntary* control.'

An important distinction, too often ignored, is the one between exercising control before conception and after. There are some people morally prepared to abide by genetically determined standards preconceptively by means of contraception, or even by sterilization, but not postconceptively by means of abortion. Others regard this distinction as arbitrary and based upon an unarguable, or at least unprovable, metaphysical assumption and belief system. There are wheels within wheels in this debate. The majority of people are realistic enough to find a pragmatic position, but there is also a whole spectrum of beliefs and "gut feelings" on the subject.

To adopt a policy of genetic control would mean giving up the game of sexual roulette, in which parents simply and blindly accept all products of conception regardless of their quality. Control means choice, of course, and choice means selection for quality. John Stuart Mill, as a champion of personal liberties, said we ought to be free to decide things for ourselves, even to die or to choose ill health, unless it hurts others.⁶ The exception means that the essence of injustice is victimizing innocent parties. In this view, carriers of bad genes are often the moral equivalents of Typhoid Mary.

Mill said, "The fact itself, of causing the existence of a human being, is one of the most responsible actions in the range of human life. To undertake this responsibility—to bestow a life which may be either a blessing or a curse—unless the being on whom it is to be bestowed will have at least the ordinary chance of a desirable existence, is a crime against that being."⁷ Genetic doom of children was not a crime in Mill's day because they could not know. Now, often, we can know.

Preventive genetic controls would interfere with the individual's right to reproduce, of course, but the whole truth is that self-determination in this case is the determination of others as well as of the self. One determines not only to have a child; it also means determining the child itself. To choose disease or hardship for others is, as Mill said, a "crime" morally speaking, and its becoming a crime legally as well cannot be far behind.

This brings us to a fairly new kind of question. Have we a moral obligation to prevent injury to *nonexistent* individuals—persons not-yet but possibly to-be? When Mill held in 1855 that "the only purpose for which power can be rightly exercised over any member of a civilized community against his will is to prevent harm to others," he had none of our new knowledge of how to control or prevent predictable harm to the unconceived and unborn. This enlarges the category of "others" who might be harmed. Many lawyers appear to restrict legal protection consciously and intentionally to *existing* persons only (i.e., to live-born individuals).[8]

As the law stands, we may voluntarily employ contraception, sterilization, and abortion to prevent a new life, as such, but the question is whether we should or must do so because the life in prospect would be diseased or defective. If we may prevent a new life simply because we do not want it, would it not be even a stronger reason that the new life to-be would or might itself not want it? Ethically, it would be absurd to contend that laws requiring marriage partners to be free of veneral disease are meant only for the protection of the uninfected partner and *not* for the sake of the children they might conceive. Genetic quality control thus raises a searching question for both moral philosophy and jurisprudence.

Most moral philosophers, like most legal philosophers, feel that the best policy is the least restrictive one consistent with a reasonable purpose and a reasonable relation of the means to the end. To endorse a policy of genetic control, therefore, raises certain subtended questions. Which disorders are grave enough to be prevented by prohibition? Here geneticists and physicians will have to put their heads together to rank-order undesired inheritances according to suffering, severity, frequency, mortality, dependency, cost, age of onset, and the like. It would be foolish to minimize the problem of constructing a rational calculus of genetic quality.

What means of control would be appropriate to various diseases? How shall we carry out a policy of mutual coercion mutually agreed upon? For example, mandatory screening, if we still leave it up to parents to choose whether to continue an affected pregnancy up to term, would not satisfy the ethical imperative. Would criteria for issuing or refusing marriage licenses do it? Would we have to have mandatory practices such as sterilization, contraception, and abortion, to back up our minimum standards? What about penalties or negative incentives to genetically responsible parenthood—perhaps taxation and levies, loss of social security benefits, schooling, custodial fees, fines, or imprisonment? In short, *how* are we to exercise responsibility?⁹

All of these questions are questions only contingently. They depend for their significance on how we answer the first and third basic questions about control itself. Ought we to be selective at all, exercising at least some measure of quality control over our reproductivity? And if so, might we ever make that control compulsory in some kinds of genetic disorder? In point of fact, only a few people (even though highly vocal) actually oppose voluntary preventive genetic control. The more biting question is about coercive control. Furthermore, if we think situationally or by case ethics, in deciding that control is justifiable, this is not by any means to say that it is *always* justifiable regardless of circumstances and variable factors. Questions of when, how, who, which, and why always arise in every category of disease, and might even arise in particular cases within a proscribed category of disease.

THE DISCUSSION

There are many people who cannot be rational about problems of quality control and human reproduction. When the question is raised, as it is bound to be more and more as time goes on, many discussants will feel uneasy; some will be threatened, a few will grow downright angry. It is important to appreciate this right from the start, not as a reason to evade the issue but as a fact to be taken into account sympathetically, or at least empathetically. As a matter of our common humanity we should understand that logical discussion is bound to be offensive to some, at least in the first stages.

Furthermore, in debates over deeply felt issues the very language we use can be a semantic trap because terms are differently conceptualized. Too often arguments are in truth mere logomachy. Words can also be tailored to slant discussion. To take a few examples: "jargon" for terminology, "gadgetry" for technology, "test tube baby" for the product of artificial insemination and *in vitro* fertilization, "manipulation" for control, "myth" for theory, "potential horrors" for risks, and "unborn baby" for fetus. We need to be on the watch for writers and speakers who practice this craft. On the other hand, such slant words may be valuable early warnings, usually of hidden or unexpressed agenda.

If we examine closely the three controversial issues we adumbrated at the beginning, and the conflicting contentions brought to bear on them, we can pick up the most important threads of this discussion. Those who claim a right to exercise control over their own lives and their children's, and thus over their own private reproduction, correctly perceive it as a right generally recognized (although not an absolute one). There are times when parents, because of their intimate role, are least able to judge what is wise or best. Those who hold to the right of the fetus to be born are assuming that fetuses as well as children are persons. A fetus, they contend, cannot plead its own case and therefore [*sic*] we have no right to decide for it without its consent, whether it is to be born or not. (Let it be noted, incidentally, that at this point the debate is really about aborting defective pregnancies, not about quality control preconceptively. Also, we should remember that many who are opposed to abortion on request do not oppose it for genetic or therapeutic reasons.)

Opponents of genetic control postconceptively (antiabortionists) further urge their prohibitionist case by insisting that genetic science is still a long way from dictating what is normal. This is beside the point, of course. First of all, geneticists readily agree that they have only started down the road to genetic knowledge. Second, basic science never dictates and it certainly does not deal in norms; that is an ethical and legal affair. Third, there are already over two thousand genetic disorders which can be diagnosed. More than sixty can be diagnosed *in utero*.

Anti-control pleaders further contend that only a child's parents may choose for it, both before and after birth. This authority (postnatally) is something the courts have already denied in various *parens patriae* decisions.[10] Ethical reasoning would raise the question for legal reasoning; if parental discretion *after birth* is properly limited for cause, why not *before birth* as well? "Pro-life" advocates have also contended that if parents disagree between themselves over the abortion of a conceptus, with the husband favoring its birth, he should prevail. (Here again, the United States Supreme Court has rejected this assertion and any laws based on it.[11])

As to a moral obligation to avoid having children with serious genetic disorders, those who assert it say we should always do what we can to realize what the courts have called "a right to begin life with sound mind and body."[12] Genetics is constantly adding to our knowledge and the means of control. In this view our responsibility grows because our control increases; it is wrong knowingly to weaken a family or the community (siblings, neighborhood, schools, hospitals, public assistance programs, and others) when we can prevent it.

The appeal of the March of Dimes is "Help Us to Prevent Birth Defects," but the way to prevent them is to prevent the birth of defective children. Anticontrol forces object that we cannot predict accurately how heavy the economic and emotional burden will be, even with the most sophisticated genetics, and therefore we ought not to make any decisions at all. This is a *non sequitur* argument from ignorance, an instance of the all-or-nothing fallacy.

Some also argue that genetic tragedies are good for those who are caught in them, teaching them patience, generosity and compassion. Usually opponents of genetic control also make a strong argument from human rights—especially to be born, to live, to reproduce, to be private and uncontrolled—yet when mention is made of a right to be born of sound mind and body, they argue that this is unrealistic, undefined, vague, impossible, and empty.

They believe, further, that it would be unjust to punish carrier parents by forbidding them to conceive and bear children with certain defects and diseases, since such parents are themselves victims. This argument assumes that parents in these tragic situations would want to pass on their bad genes and effects to their children. (Some would, of course, but only a hard core of anticontrollers.) It also assumes that "if they did it to me I can do it to somebody else." The protest that coercive control would cut across their right of self-determination is manifestly untrue: what it prevents is their determination of the lives of their children. Their objection that it interferes with their free choice is, on the other hand, patently true. This is what the debate is all about.

As to society's limiting the genetic transmission of some disorders, those in favor would contend that the community or state has an interest in preventing at least some kinds of diseases and disorders, both infectious and genetic. Assuming *arguendo* that there is a right to reproduce, a compelling social or moral interest could override that right. (Incidentally, it would be irresponsible to mandate or require diagnosis or screening for genetic disorders without requiring prevention when such traits are discovered. For example, in some provinces of Italy where thalassemia [Cooley's anemia] is endemic, applicants for a marriage license may go ahead, and marry and reproduce at will, without let or hindrance, even though the tests are positive for this recessive trait in both parties. In such cases it would be only rational not to issue the license, or to require sterilization, or at least to require antenatal tests for all pregnancies preventively. In New York too, tests of that kind may be required by law but "No application for a marriage license shall be denied solely on the ground that such tests prove positive..."[3])

Those who believe that health and the ability of citizens to carry out their fair share of ordinary social functions is vital to society regard control as a matter of contributive justice—i.e., what individuals owe to the community. In this view, parents have an obligation to uphold the social well-being; therefore, if and when society decides that some genetic faults are unacceptable, our freedom to reproduce is to that extent rightly limited. Thus the Nebraska courts have decided that "acting for the public good," citizens may be limited in their right "to bear or beget children with an inherited tendency to mental deficiency."[14]

There are far worse genetic disorders than mental deficiency, however, and preventing the victimization of potential children is as important for their own sakes as for the public good. The state has a basic interest in protecting individuals from other individuals. This is the state's oversight of commutative justice—fair play in the relations between individuals. The state imposes many statutory controls in order to protect individuals: it enforces contracts, punishes frauds, sets the quality of goods and services, detains threat makers, and the like.

Society already controls reproduction indirectly through marriage laws and through legal discrimination against children born out of wedlock; it gives its approval of healthy offspring while pitying the misbegotten. Genetic controls by coercive prevention would only apply a principle already accepted on a related level. To cope with health problems we have precedents for direct controls: in compulsory examination, quarantine, hospitalization, detention (e.g., at ports of entry), inspection of premises without a warrant, compulsory immunization, compulsory treatment for venereal disease, and preventive treatment for conditions such as neonatal ophthalmia. Why should we control the genital transmission of infectious diseases while we ignore the genetic diseases?

A related question is whether the discovery of genetic disorder by any member of a family entails a moral obligation to inform others in the family of their jeopardy. Can we remain silent without malice and culpability for what happens to innocent parents and their children? There are some who say the rights of privacy and the confidentiality of medical information cancel any obligation to share this knowledge, even with a prospective or present spouse. Would this hold, just to give one possible case, if a lethal gene were detected in an unmarried girl secretly pregnant? To warn the others in jeopardy would expose her secret.

The problem has already surfaced in areas other than genetic counseling. For example, a man loses renal function and has to go on dialysis, suffering from a genetic illness called polycystic kidney disease. Only he and his wife know what is wrong. Their son and daughter, now at the marriageable age, are ignorant of their peril (fifty percent risk) and of their children's peril, as well as the threat to those they marry. The parents refuse to tell their children the truth, fearing that it might inhibit their courtships and marriages. Should the medical staff keep mum? Ethically and legally, this is not a valid secret, since it victimizes innocent parties.[15]

Now let us look at the issues in greater depth. The presuppositions behind or beneath all such arguments, both pro and con, as well as the reasoning employed, ought to be carefully examined. Ethics, after all, is made up of (1) the values with which people approach their choices and decisions, and (2) the logic (or lack of it) with which they relate their values to their decisions. Kant very properly called ethics practical reason, because it deals with *how we decide* what we ought to do.[16]

Presuppostions play an important but often hidden part. In some disputants they are sometimes even unconscious. For example, submissively accepting the outcome of fetal life with the idea that we have to accept whatever we get, and simply enduring disordered pregnancies rather than terminating those diagnosed to be disordered, is an expression of *fatalism*. It is often tied to the notion that "nature knows best" or "we mustn't 'tamper' with nature"—opinions often reinforced by the belief that God (a) created nature, (b) has charge of natural events, especially fertilization, and (c) any human interference or initiative, as in genetic control, is an invasion of the divine monopoly, of God's prerogative. Hence the frequently heard warning against "playing God." This is a theodicy (a belief about how God is related to the world) with a long history in religious thinking and feeling.

Such fatalistic postures and taboos are, of course, opposed in logic and attitude to the principle of control, control having its own presuppositions in favor of human responsibility and the ethics of selection, choice, and decision making. In the face of natural disasters, are we "playing God" more when we do nothing at all or when we do whatever we can? Nature, after all, regularly and often aborts defective fetuses spontaneously (in more than a quarter of pregnancies); therefore, doing so for rational medical reasons is at least modeled on nature's "ethics." In truth, a good definition of medicine as a whole is "interference with natural processes."

Another presupposition of considerable influence is *individualism*. The individualist's claim of unique interest is set against the claims of the community or society.[17] Individualists find coercion by law not only unwelcome but intolerable. Opponents of genetic selectivity and control put the individual's right to reproduce ahead of all appeals to curtail it for the common good. Sometimes this individualism is based on radical egoism, sometimes on religious doctrines; in either case they come to the same thing in practice. Probably most people feel they are neither all individualist nor all communitarian, and this is probably true, but they need to understand the polarity of the concepts, even so.

Those who are willing to subordinate private desires to the social interest, if need be, back their ethical stance with the utilitarian doctrine of the greater good of the greater number, putting the well-being of the whole before the one, or of the many before the few. This "by common consent is the object of society."[18] As a humanist, the utilitarian is as concerned for only a single person as for the many, but believes that it is an imperative trade-off, *when necessary*, to sacrifice minor numbers and values for major numbers and values. This has an obvious bearing on the third basic question: Has society ever a right to intervene in human reproduction?

Still another presupposition would be about *suffering*. One argument for letting a family suffer with a diseased or defective child is that the child's suffering can be a moral plus as well as a minus; the experience, it is claimed, can ennoble all those involved, both the family and the affected individuals. A countervailing opinion is that such suffering is ennobling (when it is) and morally excusable only when it comes as a compensating factor—that to deliberately procreate a diseased or disadvantaged child for this reason is unjust, using the child as a pet rather than as a person. This argument for not preventing such births is hardly congruent with the same people's objection to selective abortion on the ground that the fetus is not consulted.

One concept with various meanings is *justice*. In the discussion of genetic control distributive justice is the main concept—sharing things out fairly. It arises in respect to a just or fair use of state supports and services, and among members of voluntary associations such as families, clubs, and churches. In the genetics problem anticontrol advocates would hold that it is fair to use up $250,000 of our economic resources per Down's victim's life, whereas procontrol advocates would deny that is. It is unfair, they contend, knowingly to produce a seriously and expensively diseased or defective child. But anticontrol spokesmen declare that the cost is simple justice and a natural or fundamental right.

The concept of *human rights* is a source of moral confusion and conflicting rhetoric. However, in spite of being conceptually precarious it is an important notion.[19] The law tries, rather awkwardly and uncertainly, to distinguish between those rights which are and those which are not fundamental, the difference being that rights of the fundamental kind are not so easily set aside, when rights conflict. In the genetics debate we are faced with claims by or for several parties: pregnant or prospectively pregnant pesons, the impregnators, their families, and society, as well as certain abstract rights such as freedom to reproduce and procreational privacy.[20]

Out of this welter it is obvious that something has to give way. As one philosopher said recently, "Rights are the stamping-ground of intuitionists, and it would be difficult to find any claim confidently asserted to a right which could not as confidently be countered by a claim to another right, such that both rights cannot simultaneously be complied with."[21] The careful formulation is that all rights are only normative: none is fundamental in the sense of undisplaceable.

In ethical terms (and in legal language) rights are relative, not absolute. In the tradition of both ethics and moral theology it is said that rights are "imperfect." This means that rights or claims of unique interest are not intrinsically valid, only extrinsically. Human needs and the variables of situations can validate or invalidate any claim. This is what the Constitution's implied power of eminent domain means in property law; the general or social interest prevails over the private interest when they conflict.

When voluntary controls cannot be relied upon, advocates of coercive control hold that as between the interests of the progenitors and a to-be misbegotten child's, the latter's interest (to avoid suffering) and society's (to avoid dependency) should prevail. They point out, furthermore, that any infringement of the progenitor's rights after conception is easily compensated by conceiving again (conceptuses are fungible), or by the availability of alternative modes of parenting (with donated gametes). In principle it is arguable that rights cease to be right and become unjust when their exercise victimizes innocent children to-be and the social fabric.

Our gonads and gametes are, strictly speaking, not our private property, in the sense of individual interest, control and possession. Biologically they are shared values. They require combination and merger with other people's genetic values (except in cloning and parthenogenesis). By and of themselves they are nothing. Testes and ovaries are, in fact, social by nature, and it would appear ethically that they should be controlled in the social interest.

It makes good sense to say that, when ethically weighed, the right to reproduce is actually only a privilege. Those who absolutize the right will retort, of course, "No. A right is a right," thus demonstrating the circularity of absolute values and rules. As seen by the rest of us, however, rights and duties are correlative ethically. The former focus on the claims of the self, the latter on the claims of others. Rights in law are like the ethical norms of right conduct in a nonabsolutistic ethics—generally but not invariably valid.

How we *determine the right course of action* when we have to make morally significant decisions is of fundamental importance. It is also probably the main source of disagreement.[22] At bottom there are only two ways to go about it. We can either follow a rule (or a ruler) of conscience, which is the *a priori* or prejudicial approach, or we can look at the facts with an open mind and calculate the consequences, the human costs and benefits, pragmatically. *Rule ethics* is in effect a policy of not deciding questions at all; if and when a rule applies it takes over and conscience is irrelevant. Negatives are taboos, positives are decrees. By contrast, relative moral judgments (decision-making ethics) will vary according to the variables in situations; values are balanced off against values. The idea is to choose the most constructive course, i.e., the one yielding a balance of benefit over risk or loss (the proportionate good). This kind of ethics truly has a place for the moral agent, so-called. It calls for choosers, not a blind following of prefabricated rules.

Those whose ethics is of the rules brand, if their rules include the right to reproduce and the right to life, often cannot tolerate putting limits on the conception or live birth of genetically diseased or defective children. For them the question is already settled ethically, and if it is believed, furthermore, that this rule is God's will, then the issue is doubly settled and predetermined. On the other hand, if we act according to *case ethics*, then it could be right either voluntarily or coercively, to limit procreation by prevention either before or after conception—if and when specified genetic diseases or defects are predictable or at risk.

For example, think of fetuses diagnosed antenatally and found to be affected. One expositor of an authoritarian ethical system allows us to let human beings die in some situations where only extraordinary means could preserve their lives, and on this ground approves of withholding the incubator from premature babies with severe genetic errors (since "extraordinary means are not usually obligatory"). This moralist's ethics also condemns abortion categorically, i.e., without discriminating among cases. It thus puts him in the odd position of being willing to let such infants die while he refuses to prevent their birth in the first place.[23] Why preventive control postnatally but not antenatally?

The hope is that only a few people are either utterly imprisoned by rules or, at the other extreme, so entirely without even generally valid guidelines that they are ethically random and unpredictable. In most cases, perhaps, people are inconsistent; they act by rules ethics sometimes, and by case ethics sometimes. Being situational lays a burden on us of decision making and moral responsibility which is both inviting and threatening. Nevertheless, ethics calls for a consistent method of making moral judgments, even though ethicists know that it is uncommon—not to say actually rare.

Case ethics is done by weighing consequences, an *a posteriori* method (as in science), in which the value standard is presumably the humanistic one, putting the well-being of persons ahead of any abstract or supernatural rules which might be cited. Many genetic counselors are inwardly torn by the ethical dilemma of their noncoercive stance ("nondirective counseling") when they and their patients have different judgments about bringing a genetically defective fetus to term.

Those who reject policies having a solid pragmatic justification often warn us that the remote consequences, if not the immediate, will add up to a balance of evil over good, if we do what they condemn on prejudicial or "principled" grounds. "If you start down that road you will end up in even worse misery and horror than the one you want to avoid." Or, "Give up even a little of your right to reproduce and you'll lose it all." A common reaction is, "This is the path the Nazis took."[24] This again is the slippery slope objection, or the entering-wedge objection.

An interesting illustration recently is an antiabortion speech by Senator Jesse Helms of North Carolina. When the Senate for the second time endorsed the use of Federal medical funds for abortion, to equalize treatment for the poor and the rich, Helms said it was the "first step to horror and tragedy" and that if this first step of what he called "killing unborn children" were taken, the next step would be to kill "the old and the feeble, the infirm and the handicapped."[25]

Scare tactics like this have some merit, however. They remind us to be careful. Sometimes remote consequences can indeed cancel out immediate benefits. The main point, however, is that the slippery slope fails to appreciate the difference between the virtue of prudence and the paralysis of fearing to take reasonable risks or accept reasonable limitations. Almost every value and policy is conceivably subject to abuse or misuse. Prudence requires us to forego foreseeable benefits if weightier undesirable side or after effects are *probable*. The "wedge" requires us, Cassandra-like, to forego such actions when the evil is only *possible*. It is a mood objection, not a reasoned argument; there is no way to verify or falsify its dire prophecies. What can we ever do that is not in some measure either ambivalent or ambiguous, or both?

Simplistic rules such as "The end does not justify the means" are ethical nonsense. Sterilizations, for example, reduce the number of unwanted pregnancies and thus the incidence of abortion. ("Prevention is the best cure.") Some people condemn both sterilization and abortion, yet they might justify one to avoid the other. One influential Catholic moralist, in a surprising concession, says: "It is my conviction that in cases of grave genetic risk sterilization is ethically more acceptable than planning selective abortion." Again, "In a society that refers now so easily to 'selective abortion' as the solution, the matter of genetically indicated sterilization should be given proper attention by the ethicists and the churches."[26]

Those who in principle oppose social control of genetic disease say that if we ever accept legal limitations on reproduction, no matter how humane the reason, the end result will be dictatorship. Then they are apt to mention Huxley's *Brave New World* and the Nazis, as evidence of what happens when biological controls are adopted. But the fact is that Aldous Huxley was a true Huxley; he believed in both biology and democracy. His fictional utopia in reverse (dystopia) was written to warn us against *political* totalitarianism—not biological.

In his preface to the 1946 edition Huxley explained that the biological nightmare in his fable resulted from a political nightmare, not the other way around, and that other controls might have been used for the purpose. In actuality, biological processes are far too slow and cumbersome to fit the urgent needs of dictators. This observation applies equally to the Nuremberg or Nazi bugaboo. The historic answer to the slippery slope is still *abusus non tollit usum*—the abuse of a thing does not bar its use.

Perhaps the most searching conflict between absolute and relative values and ethics takes shape over the sanctity (or sacrosanctity) of life versus quality-of-life evaluations. This arises in genetic control and abortion but also in treating moribund patients. Those who insist, for whatever reasons, that all life is precious regardless of conditions or potentials—a vitalistic posture which absolutizes life just because it is life—will logically oppose genetic control and abortion (although they may let a comatose patient die "naturally"). This kind of taboo or undiscriminating negative, which universalizes a prohibition, is one example of what logicians call the material fallacy of faulty generalization.

On the other side are those who would make quality choices, trying to be responsible and selective. They do not lay down blanket norms like "sterilization is always wrong" (or abortion). On this basis it is reasonable and even obligatory to obviate some genetic tragedies by sterilization before, or abortion after, conception. These things might be wrong (inhumane) in a particular case but that is the most they can assert; they cannot say "never" or "always." A quality-of-life ethic chooses the course which offers the most good, the most human benefit, and life is a value to be seen in relation to other values; at most life would only be *primum inter pares*. Thus radically are our ethics shaped by presuppositions.

It is hard, if not impossible, to wrestle with value differences as between one person and another. There is no way to prove that one value (the worth we assign to a moral or nonmoral good) is true or right while another is false or wrong. Indeed, value assertions or ascriptions are not true-false statements; they are good-evil statements. They are justifiable or unjustifiable, but they are not verifiable or falsifiable. In short, they are ethical or legal propositions, not scientific. We can disapprove of a given value but we cannot disprove it. It can be judged (assessed as to its acceptability), but that is all. This is why the end product of the legal ("judicial") process in the courts is called a judgment, as is the end product of an ethical analysis—it is not called a conclusion.

Advocates of the right to reproduce and the right to life might change their position because of data showing how deleterious reproduction is inhumane, but if so, the change would not come about by any logical necessity. It would not follow as it would where reason runs by induction and the laws of inference. Advocates of voluntary control or coercive control, and their opponents, could be equally coherent logically. They would differ not in their reasoning powers, but because of their different values.[27]

A person's values, therefore, are the key to his or her ethical position. Failure to state one's values, whether through dishonest camouflage or lack of self-knowledge, is the source of much more heat than light in ethical discourse. Furthermore, basic or first-order or cardinal values, called the *summum bonum*, or highest good, in ethics, is the seedbed and source of all the rest of a person's various derivative values. Candor about one's highest good can save a lot of time often wasted in ethical debates.

In the debate over genetic control the main moral tension lies between those for whom the highest good is compassion or humane feeling (*humanistic* ethics) and those for whom abstractions like rights and moral rules come first (*ideological* ethics). Logic leads advocates of control to contend that the principle of *non nocere* (cause no harm) in medical ethics applies as much to reproductive conduct as to clinical treatment.

We might reason pragmatically that the suffering of infants with retinoblastoma or Tay-Sachs disease or Down's syndrome or the Lesch-Nyhan disorder is sufficient reason to prevent their birth. Different diseases would presumably call for different control measures. For example, it might be decided that achondroplasia does not call for mandatory controls but Duchenne muscular dystrophy does; and so on. The courts in some cases have upheld sterilization of women incapable of taking care of children. If it is right to prevent mentally incompetent people from having children, is it not also right to prevent the birth of mentally incompetent people to begin with?

Because opponents of control give priority to other values than humaneness (perhaps the right to be left alone, or a fatalist acceptance of "typographical errors" in DNA, or whatever) they differ with procontrol forces.[28] Humanists, on the other hand, give priority to increasing the happiness and health of human beings, or reducing their suffering. In humanist ethics (and presumably in humanist jurisprudence) there is a concern to prevent harm both to those who are already born and those who are yet to be born. We protect battered children after birth; why not before? Could we call a knowing conception of a diseased baby "battery"? It is clearly an injury.[29]

Relative evaluation, pragmatic reasoning, flexible standards, humane instead of transcendental ideals, concern for human beings rather than the following of prejudicial rules—these, then, are the alternative ethical guidelines. Humanists, given their kind of ethics, see no merit in a rule of privacy or confidentiality which denies any obligation to inform relatives if we discover (by blood, serum and skin tests, or by intrauterine diagnosis) that members of one's family are at risk for a particular genetic disease. It is true that such information might cause unnecessary or false anxieties and action, and that it might be used maliciously or invite stigmatization. Nonetheless, we owe it to the extended family to share this vital information, out of humane concern. We should not keep it hidden within the nuclear family *simpliciter*.

Our bodies may be our own, but our gonads ought not to be considered as private property. We have to share our gametes if we want to reproduce ourselves. Alongside the right to privacy we have to set the right to know. There is a social need for some kind of RAPID data bank (Register to Ascertain and Prevent Inherited Diseases), even though the tension between the two values (right to privacy and right to be informed) would apply—as it does already to a number of other socially necessary controls.[30] The benefit is increased when all of those involved know how to get happier results from reproduction. The Federal Privacy Act lists fourteen exceptions to its own principle, to allow us to gain needed information.

In the humanistic outlook we might say that we are not morally obliged to have children; no law requires it, nor does any church. If we do have them, however, we are morally obliged to have the healthiest children possible, and actually ought *not* to have children if we know they are genetically doomed to grievous suffering. To reject this view is to use the right to reproduce as an admission that we are not so much upholding our own rights as we are denying the next generation their rights.

THE CONCLUSION

The conclusion here is that (1) having genetic information, we ought to set a minimum quality standard of human health and potential, for selective reproduction; (2) we ought not to bring children into the world if they will fall below the minimum standard; and (3) this minimum standard ought to be backed up by law. The third conclusion seems to be the one most widely challenged, although all three are still debated.

It should be noted, incidentally, that prudence suggests the law we want should be limited and specific, not merely a general statutory delegation of power to public health authorities.[31] At the same time, realism requires us to remember that some children will still fall below our standard; mutations, environmental insults, incomplete knowledge of genetic testing, and the like, will continue to hamper us. Nonetheless, we should do what we can, which is substantial and significant.

These conclusions presuppose an ethics of responsible control and decision making, guided by considerations of quality and social concern—considerations which give human need and happiness priority over adherence to abstract *dicta*. Each of these conclusions takes account of the new genetic sophistication now available in human reproduction—aware, of course, that a number of complex adjustments will have to be worked out. This is always the case in sociomoral growth and change. Given the interface between law and ethics referred to at the outset, the conclusions of this enquiry would seem to pose several problems for jurisprudence, involving basic questions of constitutional doctrines such as equal protection of the law, the right to due process, and freedom of conscience and religion.[32] This is an ethico-legal thicket, indeed, not to be shrugged off lightly.

One important study of the issues has agreed that there are three grounds which might be given for social control and regulation: (1) to safeguard the public health and welfare, (2) to allow a proper allocation of economic resources, and (3) to reduce human suffering.[33] (This breakdown wisely sets aside a fourth but highly problematic reason sometimes given—so-called negative eugenics.) What comes third in this list might well be put first, in the opinion of many. The most pressing concern of both parents and clinicians is the wish to spare potential children a misbegotten birth. The ethical issue is basically not statistical, but clinical. The more humane we are, the greater this concern is.

Advocates of unlimited procreation often charge that those who turn to abortion after a defective conception are indifferent to nascent life, but the charge can be turned around when the accusers refuse to prevent disasters, as in the flat prohibition of preventive abortions by church authorities following the tragic escape of dioxin gas upon villages near Milan in July, 1976.[34] We are making an assumption here, of course, that a pluralistic ethics and culture is superior to a monistic value system laid down from on high by a powerful moral authority, especially when it ignores human suffering.

It comes down in conceptual terms to "wrongful life." This emerging concept has already had its beginning in several legal cases and court judgments following the birth of diseased infants. In these cases, civil suits were brought by or on behalf of genetically diseased children when doctors had foreknowledge of their condition. "Wrongful life" is what is being avoided at the other end of life's continuum also in judicial opinions which hold that stopping treatment of moribund patients does not fall into the category of "wrongful death," a concept already well established in law. If the objection to genetic control is that the law cannot require people to do anything, or refrain from doing anything, for the sake of nonexistent individuals, we ought to reject it. A few people profess to take seriously the opinion that "no duty is conceivable except in relation to a person already in being."[35]

The law already protects future *generations* preventively by prohibiting grave insults to the environment and biosphere. A little serious reflection will show that generations consist of individuals; indeed, generations are nothing more than many individuals, protected by protecting the individuals who make them up. To injure individual descendants genetically, as when a reproductive couple procreates children knowing they will be diseased or defective, hurts the society of which they are constituent parts. Therefore, preventive legislation is fully in the public interest. Ethically (and we may suppose it to be true in jurisprudence too), we must challenge any attempt to make individuals and communities separate and mutually exclusive categories.

State enforced programs to protect the environment for the sake of both present and future generations gives the lie to any such dichotomy. On the individual scale, one court has compelled Jehovah's Witnesses to permit a blood transfusion to save a fetus, even though it had not reached the status of a Fourteenth Amendment person. There are many laws (often lacking much in the way of a scientific basis) prohibiting consanguineous marriage, to prevent possible ill effects genetically in potential children. (It seems ridiculous to prohibit consanguineous matings because of a statistical probability of bad gene combinations, while we continue to allow matings of persons definitely known to be carrying lethal genes.) What is needed is a meaningful extension of the prinicple of *parens patriae*. We ought to put the rights not to be conceived and not to be born in our bundle or normative rights. The courts have enunciated their realization that not every birth is a "happy event."[36]

The time has come to start coping with genetic control instead of sidestepping it. One eminent moral philosopher illustrates how we have failed. In a major study of justice he remarks that society should "take steps to preserve the general level of natural abilities and to prevent the diffusion of serious defects.''[37] Then he adds, "But I shall not pursue this thought here." He explains his failure to pursue it on the ground that it has not been one of "the traditional concerns of social justice." Evidently we shall have to encourage top-level thinkers to enter the new "biotic" age, getting them to bring their great gifts and commitments to bear. They are needed.

Imagine a hypothetical situation. Suppose prospective parents sought out a donor of sperm from a known carrier of isochromosome 21, with a one hundred percent risk, i.e., a certainty that the child will be affected with Down's syndrome (mongolism). Would that be wrong? If so, is it right to do it naturally, by coitus, but wrong to do it artificially, by assisted insemination? Is it not an act of "malice" in both cases? As the law stands now, couples may inflict this grievous injury at will. It would not be chance or sexual roulette since the outcome is definitely known. We do not want that kind of ethics or that kind of law.

A legal observer puts it this way: "If we approach mastery of the genetic code with careful resolve to minimize human suffering and maximize the social good, we will approach the future with assurance that, like Daedalus, we will in fact arrive safely and meet our goal. If we set out with reckless abandon and are driven by blind instinct, we surely will be corrupted and, like Icarus, fall."[38]

Objection to one line of genetic control (by means of gene "engineering") appears to undercut the whole question and render conscience and human responsibility irrelevant. This is the assertion that the general gene pool needs all its spontaneous mutations, *including even lethal genetic mutants*, and that directed mutations would undermine the genetic health of the race.[39] In short, we ought not to meddle, no matter what our reasons may be. Actually, we need not worry about having a wide enough range of probabilities; there are hundreds of thousands of loci in the human genotype, with many mutations possible in each of them. Those who want control of genetic transmissions are even accused of being unable to tolerate uncertainty. In reply we need only remark that there is no way to escape genetic uncertainty, in any case. Yet we can and should try to abate it. By voluntary contraception and abortion, Japan reduced its fetal birth defects in short order by ten percent, and Down's by forty percent.

In this study, however, we have given medical rather than eugenic reasons for genetic control. Eugenics generalizes and "statisticates" the problem away from human and personal particulars. In any case, legal or ecclesiastical prohibitions of consanguineous marriage are evidence that both state and church are already engaged in eugenic policy, through their prohibitions of incest and their tables of prohibited degrees of relationship. As a strategy to protect the gene pool it is of very uncertain utility, at best, yet how strange it is that they refuse to do it, with far more certainty, for the sake of the health and well-being of particular persons.

In the words of a distinguished American geneticist, "I would still argue for humanitarian considerations in the current generation on the grounds that we are learning more, and what we decide to do that is wrong in this generation can be reversed next generation if a wiser course of action at that time becomes apparent."[40] René Dubos puts the question in its full depth: "We are human to the extent that we are able and willing to make the choices that enable us to transcend genetic and environmental determinism, and thus to participate in the continual process of self-creation which seems to be the task and the reward of humankind."[41]

In any case, genetic improvement is due to gene pool variety, not to uncertainty. As an objection to genetic selection it is desparately speculative to say we need *all* mutations, whatever they are. It amounts only to a biological hypothesis, advanced for reasons far removed from the harsh realities of clinical medicine and genetic disease. It is not even heuristically convincing. If nature can produce desirable changes by chance mutations and adaptive selection, so can rational design produce them. It is not an either-or dilemma. Treating infectious diseases reduces them, but genetic diseases are increased by treating them; the treatment preserves the lives of those affected and through their own reproduction they spread the disease. We ought not to forget that those who insist on the right to procreate defectives are also changing the gene pool, for the worse, and since we know how to control genetic disease, at least partially, to fail to do so becomes a human "intervention" of reverse effect. Hence the far greater importance of preventive genetics than of preventive medicine. Here we have at least one solid reason for sex selection, whether carried out before or after fertilization. It will reduce transmissions of X-linked disorders.

Is this an attempt to legislate morality? It is often said that you cannot get morals by making laws. The idea behind this old saw is that laws will not work unless they reflect existing popular sentiments. The noble experiment of Prohibition is often cited. The whole story, however, is different. Civil rights laws in many parts of the United States, even though resented, have led to new behavior, which has been gradually reinforced attitudinally through the reconditioning experience of law observance. Response to the new abortion laws tells the same story.

We should be stimulating discussion of the problem. "The very rate of advance in the genetic area, and the fact that the potential social problems involve a highly esoteric body of scientific knowledge, make it difficult to expect that there will be adequate public comprehension and debate. Some means must be found to force the issues upon the public. Those means do not lie, regretfully, in simple education. It is unlikely that the public will respond to unilateral presentations of the bare facts. The public responds best to active controversy, and it is controversy and debate that should be stimulated."[42]

As a final observation, we must remember that what is ethical may not be legal, and vice-versa. Can we hope realistically that our legal and judicial system will implement controls to protect children, families, and society from the misery and burden of preventable genetic diseases? We have to turn at this point to legal analysis.

Justice White of the United States Supreme Court, with Justices Brennan and Douglas, have explained that there is no constitutional right to have children.[43] Justice Goldberg found that "...no provision of the Constitution specifically prevents the Government from curtailing the marital right to bear children and raise a family."[44] The Court further found that "...neither rights of religion nor rights of parenthood are beyond limitations."[45]

Legal concern with preventive controls of genetic disease is evident in Federal laws which provide for research, testing, and counseling for more and more specific disorders. A new law (National Genetic Disease Act) in 1976 expands coverage from sickle cell and Cooley's anemia to Tay-Sachs, cystic fibrosis, dysautonomia, hemophilia, retinitis pigmentosa, Huntington's chorea, and muscular dystrophy. The law adds, "and other genetic diseases." Yet all participation thus far has remained voluntary. What are the prospects for mandatory screening, mandatory terminations of affected pregnancies, and mandatory prevention of conception when people affected with dominant diseases and carriers of recessive diseases know their condition but refuse to restrict their reproduction?

There appears to be a strong case for voluntray control, and even for mandatory control when voluntary control does not work. But what are its prospects when it is examined as a legal question?

1. Colegrove v. Green, 328 U.S. 549, 556 (1946).

2. An actual case was Jennie Barmore in 1922. See People ex rel. Barmore v. Robertson, 302 Ill. 422, 134 N.E. 815 (1922).

3. For another survey of opinion, see an impressive paper by S.B. Twiss, "Ethical Issues in Genetic Screening: Models of Genetic Responsibility," in *Ethical, Social and Legal Dimensions for Human Genetic Disease*, ed. D. Bergsma (New York: Stratton Medical

Book Corporation, 1974), 251-258. Twiss favors voluntary control, not social or legal restraints.

4. Clifford Kirkpatrick, *Nazi Germany—Its Women and Family Life* (Indianapolis: Bobbs-Merrill, 1938).

5. This last group often shows inconsistency, e.g., they will insist on procreational privacy while also insisting on public control of fetal or other research.

6. John Stuart Mill, *On Liberty*, IV.

7. Ibid.

8. See the U.S. Supreme Court's decision in Roe v. Wade, 410 U.S. 113 (1973).

9. The term "responsible" is transitive. Its meaning shifts back and forth between culpability for what we do (blameworthiness), answerability to others for what we do (punishability), and literally an ability to respond morally (response-ability) in decisional situations.

10. E.g., McIntosh v. Dill, 86 Oklahoma 1, 205 p. 917, 925 (1922).

11. Planned Parenthood of Central Missouri v. Danforth, 428 U.S. p. 52 (July, 1976), 44 U.S.L.W. 5197 (1976).

12. In re Cavitt, 192 Neb. 712, 715, 157 N.W. 2nd 171, 175 (1968). An appeal was dismissed by the U.S. Supreme Court.

13. New York Dom. Rel., Sec. 13-aa (McKinney Suppl. 1973).

14. In re Cavitt, 192 Neb. (1968).

15. The California Supreme Court has twice found that a psychiatrist was obliged to divulge a patient's threats to kill a third party, i.e., a person other than the physician and the patient. Courts have often required ministers of religion to divulge knowledge gained in pastoral counseling or sacramental confession, in the interests of justice. (Tarasoff v. Regents of the Univ. of Calif., 118 Cal. Rptr. 129, 527 P. 2nd 553 [1974], vacated and rehearing granted No. SF 23042, March 12, 1975.)

16. Immanuel Kant, *The Critique of Practical Reason*, 1788. In practice, of course, people often make moral judgements impulsively rather than thoughtfully. Ethics, however, is the critical or rational analysis of moral opinion. Whether the moral agent acts cerebrally or viscerally is immaterial to ethics, although if the acts are compulsive they are apt to lie outside the forum of conscience.

17. An interesting up-to-date debate about this may be seen in comparing John Rawls's *A Theory of Justice* (Cambridge: Harvard University Press, 1971) with Robert Nozick's *Anarchy, State and Utopia* (New York: Basic Books, 1974). Rawls champions the common interest view, but abandons the utilitarian ground for it in favor of a more methaphysical reason.

18. W.L. Prosser, *Handbook of the Law of Torts*, Hornbook Series (St. Paul, Minn.: West Publishing Company, 1964), 15.

19. We cannot go into it here, but the verbal confusion between human rights and "right" human acts is worth a careful study. In the genetic control issue it is clear that some of the rights claimed are inconsistent with right conduct. Rights are not necessarily right. Arguing for or against rights when they are in tension or conflict is largely a contest in rhetoric.

20. Those who persist in believing that fetuses are persons would add a right of fetuses to be live-born.

21. R.M. Hare, "Abortion and the Golden Rule," *Philosophy and Public Affairs* 4 (Spring, 1975), 201-222.

22. The values and norms by which people direct their conduct make up their morals. This is properly a subject for anthropologists. Ethics is the critical examination of morals— a rational function, not descriptive but analytic.

23. Adrian M. Carr, OFM Conv., "Incubator Morally Required?" *Homiletical and Pastoral Review* 69 (April 1969), 567-568.

24. See Special Supplement, "Biomedical Ethics and the Shadow of Nazism," A conference on the Proper Use of the Nazi Analogy in Ethical Debate (April 8, 1976), *Hastings Center Report* 6 (August, 1976), 20 pp. At the conference Lucy Davidowisz, chief historian of the Holocaust, said: "I do not think we can usefully apply the Nazi experience to gain insight or clarity to help us resolve our problems and dilemmas" because it offers practically no analogy to current biomedical issues.

25. *Boston Globe*, April 26, 1976, 18.

26. B. Haering, "Genetics and Responsible Parenthood," *Kennedy Institute Quarterly Report*, (Winter, 1975) 3, 9.

27. See two papers in *Biomedical Ethics and The Law*, ed. J.R. Humber and R.F. Almeder (New York: Plenum Press, 1976). "Reproductive Rights and Genetic Disease" by L.P. Ulrich (351-360) concludes in favor of preventive control; "On Justification for Coercive Genetic Control" by T.L. Beauchamp (361-373) concludes against preventive control.

28. Garrett Hardin speaks of mutations as "typographical errors" in "DNA: The Moral Threat of Personal Medicine," *Genetic Responsibility*, ed. Mack Lipkin, Jr., and Peter T. Rowley (New York: Plenum Press, 1974), 87.

29. See M.D. Bayles, "Harm to the Unconceived," *Philosophy and Public Affairs* 5 (Spring, 1976), 292-304.

30. See Joseph Fletcher, *The Ethics of Genetic Control* (New York: Doubleday/Anchor, 1974), 194-199. This would mean expanding the services of the United States Public Health Service's Center for Disease control.

31. For example, the Illinois Domestic Relations Act (1973), sponsored by the Chicago Bar Association, providing for premarital testing for VD, added "any other diseases causing birth defects." (This is hardly a carefully considered statute.)

32. The First Amendment guarantees freedom of religious belief, but not of practice.

33. J.R. Walz and C.V. Thigpen, "Genetic Screening and Counseling: The Legal and Ethical Issues," *Northwestern University Law Review* 68 (1973), 713-726.

34. In the end, the Italian health authorities granted permission to do the abortions, suspending a prohibitory law temporarily, and physicians in the area performed them.

35. G. Tadeschi, "Liability for 'Wrongful Life'," *Israel Law Review*, (October, 1966), 513-538.

36. In re Doerr v. Villette, 74 III, App. 2nd 332, 220 N.E. 2nd 767 (1966).

37. Rawls, *A Theory of Justice*, 108.

38. G.P. Smith, II, "Manipulating the Genetic Code: Jurisprudential Conundrums", *Georgetown Law Journal* 64 (February, 1976), 697-733.

39. Marc Lappé, "Can Eugenic Policy Be Just?" in *The Prevention of Genetic Disease and Mental Retardation,* ed. Aubrey Milunski (Philadelphia: W. B. Saunders Company, 1975), 456-475.

40. J.F. Crow, "Population Perspective," in *Ethical Issues in Human Genetics*, ed. Bruce Hilton et al, (New York: Plenum Press, 1973), 73-81.

41. René Dubos, *Beast or Angel? Choices That Make Us Human* (New York: Charles Scribner's Sons, 1974), 210.

42. H.P. Green, "Mechanisms for Public Policy Decision Making," in *Ethical Issues in Human Genetics*, 393.

43. San Antonio Independent School District v. Rodriguez, 411 U.S. 1, 93 S.CT. 1278, 37 L.Ed. 2d 16 (1973).

44. Griswold v. Connecticut, 381 U.S. 479, 85 G. 1678, 1688, 14 L.Ed. 2d 510 (1965).
45. Prince v. Massachusetts, 321 U.S. 158, 166, 64 S. Ct. 438, 88 L.Ed. 645 (1944).

Ten

Abortion

Seeing how the humanhood and abortion issues surface everywhere in biomedical ethics, I want to take a more sharply focused look at both questions.

For some of us "human nature" is fixed, a given entity; for others, the human organism and psyche are malleable and adaptable. T.E. Hulme said, "Man is an extraordinarily fixed and limited animal whose nature is absolutely constant."[1] To the contrary, Ashley Montagu explains that babies are not born with a human nature, only with more or less capability of *becoming* human.[2] In the same vein the Spanish philosopher Ortega y Gasset concluded that people have no nature; they have only their histories.[3]

Actually, we have to ask whether it is human life we put first or *personal* life? If it is personal human life, then our first-order concern is with certain qualities and capacities, not just human life as such. In short, may we use 'a human life' and 'a person' interchangeably? The philosopher Henry David Aiken calls it "fetishism" to believe that a fetus is already a person. But is he justified in saying so?[4] This question is of the greatest practical importance in making decisions about such matters as the terminally ill and when to let the patient go, in dealing with irreversible coma, and whether we ought to "save" what are called monsters at birth. When we quote the Socratic maxim Know thyself, what *is* the self, the person? Not to know what we mean by these key terms is simply to flounder around when we talk about moral decisions.

Abortion provides a test. Ethically the core issue is whether an embryo or fetus is a human being, and if so, in what sense we call it that. How we assess the morality of abortion follows from how we answer this question.

For example, a Catholic lawyer says flatly, "One person's freedom to obtain an abortion is the denial of another person's right to live."[5] He believes that a fetus is a person or has a person's rights. There is no argument, of course, about a human fetus being of the species *Homo sapiens*; it is easily recognizable biologically. Nor is there any question of its being alive. Cell division is proceeding. But what about claims of personhood or humanhood for a fetus? If every human fetal organism is a person, and if we think it is immoral to end such forms of human life unnecessarily—at least when self-defense or the common security is not at stake—we will logically look upon abortion at will as immoral. If, on the other hand, we do not regard uterine life as human in the sense of a personal being, we will not believe its termination is "murder"—that is, we won't see it as taking the life of an innocent person. The nonpersonal view of fetuses fits in with the morality of elective abortion or abortion on request, as well as with therapeutic abortion for medical reasons.

The ethical issue is dramatized in a truly tragic situation in a Nazi concentration camp.[6] A Romanian woman doctor secretly aborted three thousand Jewish women in the camp because if the medical report showed them to be pregnant, they would be incinerated—sent to the ovens. If we believe that a fetus is a person, it would follow that the doctor, by killing three thousand human beings, saved three thousand others and prevented the murder by the Nazis of all six thousand. On the nonpersonal basis we would say only and quite calmly that three thousand persons were rescued from a terrible death. (The United States Congress agreed with the latter interpretation. The doctor was admitted to residence and citizenship in America as a war hero.)

The most basic issue is whether a fetus is a person or not. This in turn poses the question, What's the *essence* of a person? Along with it goes the related question, When does this essential element emerge, whatever it is? The question of what a person is hinges on whatever is held to be the essence. There would be room for some variety of opinion on additional factors, the other things which make for the fullness or optimum of a person. The decisive problem is to identify the essential thing, the *sine qua non*, that without which there is no person. And to find this key is to get pretty close to answering the question about "when" a person is.

What are the factors or components which people have suggested is the essential one? There are three of them, basically. Some argue that life is the essential element in a person's being; whenever and as long as we are alive, as long as life is present, they say, a human organism is a person. This would mean that a person exists at fertilization, when growth gets started, and continues to exist through the whole complex biological continuum. Indeed, *before* fertilization oöcytes and sperm are "alive." Death is not complete until the cessation not only of bodily functions but even of cell activity. This opinion identifies the person with life, making the two coexistent or even one and the same. It is the doctrine behind recent agitation to prohibit tests and research with live abortuses, even though there is no possibility of the fetus surviving and even though the knowledge to be gained by obstetricians and pediatricians could save the lives or health of many children yet to be born. It is a radical and sad consequence of an absolute sanctity-of-life ethics.

A second notion is that, not life, but the soul makes a person. In this camp we find two different ideas about the soul's entrance into the living tissue. While they both agree that it enters somehow before the birth of the individual, some guess or believe that the soul or *animus* enters after conception, probably in the second trimester ("delayed animation") and others guess it enters with fertilization ("immediate animation")—thus coinciding, in the latter case, with the *life* theory. An obvious absurdity of this latter doctrine is that it means the soul or person of identical twins has been split in two, since after fertilization they separated from a common cell mass or single fertilized ovum. Triplets, quadruplets, and so on, add to the absurdity of the ensoulment-at-fertilization doctrine. Aristotle, Augustine, and Aquinas held to the late ensoulment theory and therefore justified abortion, at least in the first trimester; Tertullian, the great heretic, declared for the fertilization idea, and his opinion finally became the official Catholic teaching in 1869, when abortion was condemned at any stage. (The papacy has never actually said when the soul is infused; rather, it has decreed that people must play it safe by acting *as if* the soul were infused at fertilization.)

The third opinion is that the essence of a person is reason, the rational function, the *ratio*. In this view everything depends on the mental capability of the individual. This is not to say that reason is everything; feeling is an important part of mental function, too. But without intelligence the feeling alone is subhuman. The cerebral has to undergird the visceral. Before cerebration comes into play, or when it is ended, in the absence of the synthesizing or *thinking* function of the cerebral cortex, the person is nonexistent; or, put another way, the life which is functioning biologically is a nonperson. This nonpersonal condition can be seen both in the protoplasm at the start of life and in the "human vegetable" which is sometimes all that remains at the end.

Humans without some minimum of intelligence or mental capacity are not persons, no matter how many of their organs are active, no matter how spontaneous their living processes are. If the cerebrum is gone, due to disease or accident, and only the mid-brain or brainstem is keeping autonomic functions going, they are only objects, not subjects—they are *its*, not *thous*. Just because heart, lungs, and the neurologic and vascular systems persist, we cannot say a *person* exists. Noncerebral organisms are not personal.

The Harvard Medical School's *ad hoc* committee accepted the "brain death" definition, but it is too undiscriminating. So is the Kansas statute modeled on it, and the recent (1972) ruling of the Italian Council of Ministers. It is not the death of the *brain* that counts. What is definitive is the absence of cerebration or "mind" even though other brain functions continue. A human vegetable is not a person, not truly a human being. It goes without saying, of course, that the loss of the cerebral function must be determined to be irreversible.

According to this third view, perhaps something like a score of twenty on the Binet scale of I.Q. would be roughly but realistically a minimum or base line for personal status. Obviously a fetus cannot meet this test, no matter what its stage of growth.

Nor can a fetus have any of the other traits that make for the full *humanum* or personal quality, such as curiosity, affection, self-awareness and self-control, memory, purpose, conscience—none of the distinctive transbiological indicators of personality. The fetus-is-a-person doctrine is of necessity the most argumentative one because it has to defend an arbitrary assertion. The nonpersonal view is under no such strain. It asserts nothing not in evidence, and therefore it really does not have to be defended or make a case for itself.

Antiabortion agitators often say, "Well, anyway, there is a *potential* in the fetus for all of these things that make up a person; for example, the morphon or rudimentary physical basis of mind is present by the eighth month." This is tantamount to admitting that a fetus is in fact *not* a person. And to argue (which is what this is—*arguing*) that the potential is the actual is like saying that an acorn is an oak or a promise is its fulfillment or a blueprint is a house. The "as if" argument is a prolepsis which tries to wipe out the vital difference between what is and what could be. Thomas Aquinas was at least right to distinguish between human life *in potentia* and *in sit* (actual) and to assign personal status only to the latter, after several months' gestation.

The plain inescapable fact, as a chemist might say, is that we have no litmus paper test for the presence of a person. Jean Rostand, the French biologist, puts it this way: "It must be said that these differing opinions are held by people who are equally sincere, have the same level of morality, and sometimes even profess comparable philosophical doctrines."[7] Any attempt to impose a single "doctrine" on those who do not share it is ethically intolerable. We are driven to admit that, if anybody wants to believe a fetus is a person at conception or whenever it is "ensouled," he is entitled to. It is a kind of mental Mexican stand-off.

The only possible moral test of these rival views lies in their consequences. When beliefs or nonempirical opinions, neither of them being falsifiable, contradict or clash with each other, the only possible way to choose between them morally is in terms of their consequences if they are followed out logically in practice. The one which results in greater good for people is the correct one. On this basis there is an open and shut case for abortion, obvious and overwhelming; it can be justified very often, sometimes for reasons of human health, sometimes for reasons of human happiness.

Furthermore, the question of *when* the person comes into existence, the timing, has never found any general agreement or any convincing evidence favoring one opinion over others. In the past people have argued variously that this event or "moment" is at (1) fertilization, (2) the blastocyst or implantation stage, (3) the first heartbeat, (4) the phenomenon of "kicking" or "quickening," (5) viability—when the fetus might maintain its life outside the womb (sometime in the third trimester), and finally (6) birth. Here, too, we have no litmus paper test, no diagnostic criteria. When the Grand Mufti of Jerusalem says the "moment" is the 120th day of pregnancy, like the theologians who used to say it was forty days in the case of males and eighty days for females, we can only try to keep a straight face.

The most sensible opinion is Plato's, that a fetus becomes a person at birth—after it is expelled or drawn from the womb, its umbilical cord is cut, and its lungs start to work. This has been the opinion held down through the centuries in the common law tradition. It was not until the nineteenth century that abortion was for the first time made a crime—although, be it noted, only against the state because of the supposed loss of a much needed citizen, soldier, or worker. Crowded subways and expressways, growing lists of hard-core unemployment in the midst of highly productive industrial and agricultural machinery—these things make the "public interest" of a century ago archaic.

Later on, some groups began to claim that abortion is a crime against the *fetus* as well as against the state, with the result in America that new laws began to prohibit termination of pregnancy for any reason other than to save the woman's life or, in a few states, her health. In spite of these new statutes, however, no prosecutor has ever returned an indictment for murder in any abortion case before the courts. In cases of miscarriage no birth certificates are made out, and abortions of such fetal tissue are not entered into the vital statistics. Pregnant women traveling abroad have not been required to carry two passports, one for themselves and one for the fetus. Miscarried embryos at a primitive stage are not baptized.

On and on we could go, pointing out similar lapses or discrepancies between what people preach and what they practice. In 1972, before the Supreme Court's decision in January 1973, spokesmen for the Right to Life Movement carried around a fairly fully formed human organism, superficially, and displayed it for the shock effects ("homunculus reaction") on uncritical and impressionable people in audiences. When they were asked if the fetus had been baptized or entered into the birth statistics, christened with a name, and "Why hasn't this child, as you call it, been buried with respect"—their replies were only mumbles, not even clear words.

For some time legislators and courts have been revamping those Victorian laws in a return to the main tradition, to the view that a fetus is not a person or what American lawyers call a "Fourteenth Amendment person." The chief reason for the postnatal definition of a person in the law is that any other doctrine is necessarily only a matter of private faith or belief, and it is morally unjust to impose private beliefs upon others who do not share them. To do so violates the First Amendment of the Constitution which guarantees religious freedom and freedom of thought.

The United States Supreme Court on January 22, 1973, declared that it is unconstitutional for any state to forbid abortion in the first trimester, which only reaffirms the historic position of Western civilization. The question *when* a pregnancy should be terminated for health reasons is a medical one, the Court explained, and not a proper government function.

This decision knocked down restrictive statutes in forty-six of the fifty states of the Union. It means that freedom of abortion may not be regulated in the first six or seven months—but after the first six months the state would be *allowed* but not *required* to limit abortions. The Court rejected any assignment of *personal* status to the fetus at any stage, and allowed only that a government might find a public interest in *potential* human life, and even then not until the fetus has become capable of survival independent of the maternal body. It has no rights.

In any case, in the last analysis it remains the patient's choice, on the principle of consent, as in any other medical or surgical treatment. This freedom of choice coerces no physician into doing an abortion nor any patient into having one. The Court did not enter into the ethical-moral question, it is true; yet by finding for the nonpersonal view of fetal life, it put the focus where it really belongs, and more profoundly affected the moral issue than any court judgment for hundreds of years.

Only if we can decide where we stand on these issues can we decide where we stand on the morality of terminating pregnancies. In practical policy terms, there are four positions to choose among, and our choice will depend on what we decide about the status and quality of the fetus. (1) We can condemn abortion altogether, or at most only justify it to save the pregnant woman's life. (2) We can favor a limited permissiveness to prevent ill health, to prevent defective babies, or to prevent the product of rape or incest. This is a policy of compulsory pregnancy but with escape clauses. (3) We can approve of abortion for any reason prior to the ability to survive outside the womb—possibly on the grounds of social needs or some question of justice, although these grounds are not so apparent as they were when we lacked enough labor power and needed lots of soldiers. (4) We can oppose any and all forms of compulsory pregnancy, making the ending of pregnancies, like their beginning, a private or personal matter.

If we adopt the sensible view that a fetus is not a person, there is only one reasonable policy, and that is to put an end to compulsory pregnancy. The ethical principle is that pregnancy when wanted is a healthy process, *pregnancy when not wanted is a disease*—in fact, a venereal disease. The truly ethical question is not whether we can justify abortion, but whether we can justify compulsory pregnancy. If our ethics is of the humane brand we will agree that we cannot justify it, and would not want to.

Many sensitive people who support abortion in principle nevertheless see it as a sad, even tragic, action. In this view abortion is a reason for regret, but not for remorse or moral guilt. To deplore abortion is *a fortiori* a strong reason to advocate contraception. To condemn both—both the termination and the *prevention* of unwanted pregnancies—is an antisexual and inhumane morality. (This is what the official Catholic teaching does, except that it allows "natural" birth control by "rhythm," which helps us to understand the grass roots revolt of Catholics who defy their church's ban on contraceptives and sterilizations.)

1. T.E. Hulme, *Speculation: Essays in Humanism and the Philosophy of Art* (New York: Harcourt, Brace & Company, 1946), 11.

2. Ashley Montague, *Sex, Man and Society* (New York: G. P. Putnam's Sons, 1969).

3. José Ortega y Gasset, *Man and People* (New York: W. W. Norton & Company, 1957).

4. Henry David Aiken, "Life and the Right to Life," in *Ethical Issues in Human Genetics*, ed. B. Hilton, et al. (New York: Plenum Press, 1973), 182.

5. J. Noonan, ed. *The Morality of Abortion* (Cambridge: Harvard University Press, 1970), xvii.

6. See Joseph Fletcher, *Situation Ethics* (Philadelphia: Westminster Press, 1966), 38.

7. Jean Rostand, *Humanly Possible* (New York: Saturday Review Press, 1973), 88.

Eleven

Infanticide

Obviously the ethics of abortion runs close to the ethics of infanticide. Antiabortion agitators commonly raise the specter of infanticide: "First they want to kill little babies before they are born; next thing, they'll try to kill them *after* they're born." If fetacide is morally licit, why not infanticide?

The question whether infanticide is ever justifiable, and if so *when*, can be better appreciated if we begin by locating infanticide on the total map of induced death, that is to say, of death humanly intended and contrived. Therefore I shall first look at the moral variants in a spectrum of the different ways we might take to induce death, and then focus on infanticide in particular.

In what follows we will be looking primarily at dying when it is chosen or elected in the sick room, which might be called medical euthanasia. I will prescind from such practices as vendetta, military life-taking, capital punishment, mortal risk-benefit choices, and other ways of assuming control over life and death—other kinds of human decisions not to leave death to "natural" causes. *The Oxford English Dictionary* defines euthanasia (literally 'good death' or what medieval philosophers called *bene mori*) this way: "In recent use: the action of inducing a gentle and easy death." Several variables arise as between medical and nonmedical situations, even though the constants are equally important. In our present society, however, the problem is more commonly posed in the context of medical care and treatment.

The moral problems of suicide and allocide are, of course, not new. Nevertheless, they are taking a new shape recently because of advances in medical capabilities, especially in resuscitation and life-support technologies. Once upon a time the typical problem in serious, life-threatening illnesses was to find a way to prolong life, but often now the problem is how long and how much to do so, particularly when we find we are prolonging dying rather than living, "saving" biological life at the expense of human life.

LOCATING INFANTICIDE

My premise will be that induced death, as such, may not be condemned categorically, and that truly rational ethical issues only arise when responsible moral agents set about determining answers to operational questions—who, why, what, when, and how. It is unreasonable ethically to say that all acts of euthanasia are wrong, just as it would be to say that none is.

Another premise is that what is good and right for a person when he does it for himself, e.g., suicide, is just as good and right when it is done for him by proxy (i.e., allocide). Thus the English law which decriminalizes self-administered euthanasia but continues to outlaw it when it is carried out by others such as physicians, nurses, paramedics, or a member of the family, at the subject's request or with his agreement, is logically untenable.

The most significant ethical discrimination we make when we evaluate intended and induced dying ("elective death") is between voluntary and involuntary cases. This would at least be true for those with whom freedom of choice is a highly important element of personal integrity—a first-order value. The "right to die" is therefore taken ordinarily to mean one's right to choose one's own death, rather than any right (at least ordinarily) to choose death for somebody else.

Voluntary dying is chosen consciously by the subject, whether in the event or prior to it. An example would be fulfilling the wishes of patients that treatment be stopped when to do anything more would be fatuous. Their wishes might be expressed either at that time or recorded earlier in a living will. Involuntary dying would be exemplified by an accident victim's death on the operating table, or stopping a comatose patient's treatment because to continue would be pointless and cruel—the decision being made without the patient's consent and without any knowledge of his preference, past or present. The difference hangs on the factor of consent.

Euthanasia, however, poses not one but four critical distinctions. Its form may vary not only as to (1) consent (voluntary or involuntary), but also as to (2) whether the method used to end the patient's life is by a positive act or by omitting life-preserving treatment (direct or indirect), (3) whether the agent of the action is the subject himself or somebody else (active or passive), and (4) whether the patient's condition is terminal or nonterminal—i.e., whether or not death has been determined to be imminent.

Direct euthanasia is death induced by doing something that entails the patient's death as an immediate consequence. Instances would be the patient's taking a highly toxic drug such as potassium cyanide, or the physician's administering it, or somebody's removing an endotracheal tube from a patient with pulmonary arrest. Euthanasia is indirect when something is done which foreseeably results in death as a "subsequence" but not the direct consequence. Such would be a patient's refusal to eat, or disconnection by him (or another) of intravenous inserts for hyperalimentation (i.e., starving the patient to death). This direct-indirect distinction has to do, in short, with whether the relation between cause and effect is immediate or not, i.e., whether the foreseeable result of the action follows at once from the act or only after a series of effects set in train by the primary action.

A pathetic case illustrating the direct-indirect phase of infanticide occurred some years ago at the Johns Hopkins Hospital in Baltimore. It has had a wide follow-up discussion, based on a film about it circulated for teaching purposes. A newborn had all the stigmata of Down's syndrome, and the parents therefore refused consent to the corrective surgery needed to remove a duodenal atresia and thus to open up the infant's food tract and save it from death.

The physicians in charge believed that direct euthanasia is wrong, but that doing it indirectly, though undesirable, was morally tolerable. Hoping that the newborn would die of dehydration and starvation in three or four days, they wheeled it off into a corner where it lay dying for fifteen days, not three or four. Some form of direct termination would have been far more merciful as far as the infant, nurses, parents and some of the physicians were concerned. In that case, indirect was morally worse than direct—if, as I and most of us would contend, the good and the right are determined by human well-being. Indirect euthanasia did no good at all in that case, but lots of evil.

The third distinction, between active and passive, has to do with whether an act of euthanasia is done by the patient or by somebody else. It is active when the subject (patient) does it, for example, by taking an overdose of a barbiturate or opiate. It is passive when another person does it for the subject, whether directly (e.g., closing down a patient's lungs with a specific for pulmonary paralysis) or indirectly (e.g., removing the support provided by a respirator). We have already suggested that there is no ethical difference between active and passive ways of inducing death. The only difference is in the agent, which makes it suicide or allocide, but this is instrumental, not intentional. Either way the patient's death is the end being sought, whether the patient or some other person brings it about. If the patient's release from an irreversibly painful and hopeless existence is contrived for him instead of by him, no onus lies on the agent unless it lies on the patient too.

By the same reasoning, direct and indirect euthanasia are morally alike, on a par. As I will contend later, it is morally evasive and disingenuous to suppose that we can condemn or disapprove positive acts of care and compassion, but in spite of that approve negative strategies to achieve exactly the same purpose. Kant was on sound ground to insist that, if we will the end, we will the means. Purposive acts of commission are morally no different from acts of omission that have the same goal. A decision not to open an inperforate anus in a trisomy-18 newborn is "mercy killing" as surely as if a poison pellet were used. Not eating is suicide as surely as jumping off the Eiffel Tower; it just takes longer.

Our fourth and last distinction is between terminal and nonterminal cases. A patient is terminal if he is going to die of his present condition no matter what treatment is given. An example would be the man with amyotrophic lateral sclerosis in Dr. I. S. Cooper's novel, *It's Hard to Leave While the Music's Playing.*[1] A nonterminal case would be one in which death would not be expected from any present pathology, e.g., a person who hangs himself because his life, as such, does not seem worth living.

In short, euthanasia has significantly different forms. It may be voluntary or involuntary, direct or indirect, active or passive, a response to terminal illness or to some other condition. A number of combinations and permutations of these variances is to be met with every day in the realities of dying, as human beings strive to control dying for human or humane reasons. Some of these differences, however, are without much if any ethical weight.

INFANTICIDE

Infanticide is the induced death (euthanasia) of infants. Because of their various deficits, when death comes to infants it is necessarily involuntary. Whether it comes naturally or by human design, it happens without the subject's knowledge or consent. Knowledge and consent are impossible—as impossible for neonates as for fetuses when abortion is considered. It is reasonable, indeed, to describe infanticide as postnatal abortion, which is what it obviously was in the South Pacific when Robert Louis Stevenson visited the atolls and found that the Polynesians practiced infanticide when newborns showed disabling birth diseases and defects. (Theirs was a situation of radically scarce resources, both economic and medical, and Stevenson's initial revulsion was set aside after a period of observation.)

Furthermore, infanticide is passive. An infant cannot put an end to its own life. This makes it allocide, not suicide. Its variables are only (1) with respect to the choice of direct or indirect means, and (2) whether it is done within the context of terminal illness or some other adverse state.

Some writers have argued that a fetus is a person as truly as an infant is, and that therefore both abortion and infanticide are unjust killing (murder). This argument has as its premise the rule that persons (human beings) ought never to elect or be elected to die by human initiatives. This universal negative or prohibition implies that death must always be imposed nonhumanly by God or nature or some other cosmic arbiter. It is a position with which we are familiar in classical Catholic moral theology and Protestant ethics (although not all theologians defend it), and in "pro-life" propaganda.[2] Paul Ramsey has defended this view.[3] I would support the opposite position, i.e., that both abortion and infanticide can be justified if and when the good to be gained outweighs the evil—that neither abortion nor infanticide is as such immoral. John Fletcher has tried to establish a middle position, arguing for the licitness of abortion but against infanticide.[4] He gives three reasons why infants are different from fetuses and should be differently treated: (1) a neonate has a separate existence, (2) tends to arouse parental feelings of attachment, and (3) is treatable. (Each of these things, however, is true of fetuses too.)

Another ground for opposing infanticide has been chosen by E-H. W. Kluge.[5] His major premise is his belief or metaphysical assertion that an infant is a person, which he defines as any individual with not only an actual but a *potential* capacity for human self-awareness. His contention is that persons, *qua* persons, have a right to live—and that ethically this right may not be abridged. Because, in his opinion, a "structural potential" exists in fetuses (he fails to discriminate those cases in which the potential is not present), he assigns personal status to both fetuses and infants. He concludes: "Therefore infanticide is—to say the least—morally reprehensible. In fact, it is murder." (This appears to be an instance of the fallacy of the potential, i.e., arguing by prolepsis that the potential is the actual.)

Here we come to the crucial issue. Do persons, however defined, have an absolute or unqualified right to live? The courts have never found one, nor has jurisprudence. So-called human rights, as a term much employed in political rhetoric, are certain moral claims (e.g., to privacy, to property, liberty, and the like) which are ordinarily or commonly conceded. Street talk about "rights" ("I have a right to" such things as relief checks, free parking, health care, education, old age benefits, or whatever) means nothing more than an expression of belief, well- or ill-founded, that people *ought* to have certain things. However, all these claims are only relatively valid, whether they are or are not constitutionally formulated. At best they are only "prima facie." They are relative and not absolute for the sufficient reason that they can and often do cut across each other. Ethical problems are, when thoroughly examined, problems of relative choice among competing values or "goods," and to posit values at all entails priorities for making risk-benefit and gain-loss judgments. Hence the relativity of rights.

Kluge's real sting is in his tail. Not until the very last sentence of his discussion of infanticide does he come out of the closet and declare openly, "And if it is argued that this [condemnation of infanticide] depends on the further assumption that there are absolute values, I must unabashedly admit that this is something I hold to be the case."[6]

This means, if it means anything, that the life of persons, which he believes infants and fetuses to be, has an absolute value that cannot be weighed in any moral scales relative to other competing values and dysvalues. It means that life, as such, is sacrosanct and taboo, no matter how much suffering and tragedy and deprivation might be the price.[7] Given this as his "bottom line" he (Kluge) could not cope with the kind of decision making needed for an infant with 94.5 percent full-thickness, 92 percent total-body burns, and irreversible lung damage from smoke inhalation. Or, again, how could he make a judgment ethically about an infant with spina bifida cystica, plus a meningomyelocele and meningeal infection already widespread? Or an infant born with retinoblastoma after slipping through the antenatal screen, and postoperative diagnosis shows that the surgical removal of its eyes has not stopped the spread of cancer?

If the life of these infants, such as it is, is sacrosanct as far as human initiatives are concerned, they would have to suffer—according to the taboo ethic—until they died "naturally" or until "God called them" out of life. If life is absolutely good, unconditionally good, we cannot talk about quality of life, since in common use the phrase requires us to be open to judging the quality of life itself, as well as making quality judgments on things within the ambiance of life. As the Jesuit theologian

R. A. McCormick once put it, ethical reasoning collapses when anybody says, "There is no such thing as a life not worth living."[8]

The rejoinder to Kluge and others like him is that they have misplaced the debate. Careful and candid analysis will show that deciding whether and when an infant is a person is not the determinative question. The right one is, "Can a person's life ever be ended ethically?"* It all turns on the issue of whether the value of a human life is absolute or relative. It is this metaethical question which lies at the heart of the disagreement about infanticide. We could accept Kluge's thesis that fetuses are persons, and still justify both abortion and infanticide in some cases, because, in a given case, to prolong life would be to engender more evil than good. This tragic situation occurs frequently in perinatal medicine, even though its frequency is not great statistically. It is Kluge's second premise (that we may not take a person's life) which is rejectable, whether or not we accept his first premise (that fetuses and infants are persons). As an absolute taboo he cannot justify this on humane or humanistic grounds. It must presumably be supported by a cosmic authority, God or Mother Nature, established by revelation or metaphysics. (Whatever it is, he keeps it secret and undeclared.)

Pediatricians or others who would sometimes justify letting a newborn die, or even helping a newborn to die, would do so on value grounds. Life itself would be only one value among values, even though a high-order one, and therefore some infants' lives (like some lives in any other age group) might properly be sacrificed on the principle of proportionate good. (No undeclared premises are hiding behind the discussion in this essay, by the way. It is based on ethical relativism—i.e., situational or contextual relativism, not cultural relativism. This is my mode of approach to the ethics of induced death in general and infanticide in particular.)

To contend there are cases in which it is good and therefore right to induce the end of a person's life obviously assigns the first-order value to human well-being, either by maximizing happiness or minimizing suffering. This view assigns value to human *life* rather than to being merely *alive*, and holds it is better to be dead than to suffer too much or to endure too many deficits of human function. In this mode of ethical reasoning the criterion of obligation is caring or kindness or loving concern—various terms have been used to denote it.[9] Its basic value stance is that we ought to do whatever promotes well-being and reduces suffering, and therefore if ending a life is judged to do so, so be it.

*Kluge compromises his taboo by allowing one exception—killing in self-defense.

William Frankena has classified my ethics as "modified act agapism," which simply means that loving concern for human beings comes first, before rules of conduct.[10] As Frankena shows, it is a form of utilitarianism and consequentialist ethical decision making. The only "rule" it follows consistently is to do whatever offers the most human benefit, and on this basis we would sometimes save lives, sometimes end them (directly or indirectly, actively or passively).

In another place, citing various philosophical discussants, Frankena rashly and arbitrarily says that Henry Sidgwick, William Temple, and I all assume the belief in the "sanctity of life" means holding life to be absolute and inviolable, but in fact all three of us accept the distinction Frankena draws between *absolute* respect for life (not, however, sanctifying it) and "qualified respect for human life"—which last Frankena and the rest of us endorse, all alike.[11]

Loving concern ("*agape*") is a standard of good and evil which could be validated in either a theistic or a humanistic belief system. A theist might, of course, believe that God forbids infanticide by a rule, perhaps along with other things such as adultery or baking bread on Sundays. On the other hand, he might believe that the divine will or commmand is only that we do the most loving thing possible in a given situation, leaving it to the moral agent to decide what that is. Likewise, a humanist might decide that ending infants' lives is in general inhumane and therefore ought never to be done (as with some rule utilitarians),[12] or he might hold instead that we should seek to optimize human well-being in every case, thus sometimes allowing for infanticide (as in act utilitarianism).

If one's standard of the good is human well-being, and one's duty or obligation is to seek to increase it wherever possible, with a consequent willingness to save lives sometimes and end them sometimes, then it will follow that infanticide is acceptable (sometimes). If one's standard is a divine will or other cosmic authority (e.g., Natural Law) one could still accept infanticide, depending on whether the divine will is believed to be expressed in universal and absolute rules (such as we find in revealed codes), or in a general command to be loving (beneficent, kind, humane, et cetera), with flexibility as to the variables in particular cases.

In fact, differences between religious ethics and autonomous ethics do not determine the issue of infanticide. The only real issue is whether concern for persons in hopeless misery ranks higher or lower than taboo.

1. I.S. Cooper, *It's Hard to Leave While the Music's Playing* (New York: W. W. Norton and Company, 1977).

2. For a notably fair account of the ethical issues, yet firmly favoring the established teaching, see Leonard J. Weber, *Who Shall Live?* (New York: Paulist Press, 1977), 53-72.

3. Paul Ramsey, "Abortion," *The Thomist* 37 (1973), 174-226.

4. John Fletcher, "Abortion, Euthanasia, and Care of Defective Newborns," *The New England Journal of Medicine* 292 (January 9, 1975), 75-78.

5. Eike-Henner W. Kluge, *The Practice of Death* (New Haven: Yale University Press, 1975), 207-209.

6. Later on Kluge says that, although there are absolute rules, nobody has yet identified them, and this he promises to do at some future time. Ibid., 242-244.

7. As the historian, Barbara Kellum, and others have shown, even in the religious era of medieval England, infanticide, like abortion, was regarded as only a venial sin, not mortal. Thomas of Cobham's penitential said that if an infant was disposed of by its mother's own hand it was a venial sin equal to overlaying, as was a refusal to nurse an infant. For a summary account, see Catherine Damme, "Infanticide: the worth of an infant under law," *Medical History* 22 (January, 1978), 1-24.

8. R.A. McCormick, "To Save or Let Die: the Dilemma of Modern Medicine," *Journal of the American Medical Association* 229 (July 8, 1974), 172-176.

9. Bentham and Mill called it utility. Martin Kohl calls it "reasonable kindness" in his *The Morality of Killing* (London: Peter Owen, 1974). In my own language it is called loving concern (*Situation Ethics* [Philadelphia: Westminster Press, 1966]).

10. William Frankena, *Ethics* 2nd ed. (Englewood Cliffs, New Jersey: Prentice-Hall, 1973), 36, 55-57.

11. "The Ethics of Respect for Life," in *Respect for Life in Medicine, Philosophy and Law,* by O. Temkin, W. K. Frankena, and S. H. Kadish (Baltimore: Johns Hopkins University Press, 1976), 32-33.

12. Rule utilitarianism could theoretically set up an opposite norm or rule, i.e., that it is *right* to practice infanticide in certain kinds or classes of situations, but it would still be a rule: the moral agent would not be free to judge for or against what the rule stipulated— would not, in other words, be morally responsible.

Twelve

Euthanasia

It is harder morally to justify letting somebody die a slow and ugly death, dehumanized, than it is to justify helping him to escape from such misery. This is the case at least in any code of ethics which is humanistic or personalistic, i.e., in any code of ethics which has a value system that puts humanness and personal integrity above biological life and function. It makes no difference whether such an ethics system is grounded in a theistic or a naturalistic philosophy. We may believe that God wills human happiness or that man's happiness is, as Protagoras thought, a self-validating standard of the good and the right. But what counts *ethically* is whether human needs come first—not whether the ultimate sanction is transcendental or secular.

What follows is a moral defense of human initiatives in death and dying. Primarily I mean active or direct euthanasia, which helps the patient to die, not merely the passive or indirect form of euthanasia which "lets the patient go" by simply withholding life-preserving treatments. The plain fact is that indirect or negative euthanasia is already a *fait accompli* in modern medicine. Every day in a hundred hospitals across the land decisions are made clinically that the line has been crossed from prolonging genuinely human life to only prolonging subhuman dying; and when that judgment is made, respirators are turned off, life-perpetuating intravenous infusions stopped, proposed surgery canceled, and drugs countermanded. So-called Code 90 stickers are put on many record-jackets, indicating "Give no intensive care or resuscitation."

Arguing pro and con about negative euthanasia is therefore merely
flogging a dead horse. Ethically, the issue whether we may let the patient
go is as dead as Queen Anne.

Straight across the board of religious traditions there is substantial
agreement that we are not morally obliged to preserve life in *all* terminal
cases. (The religious-ethical defense of negative euthanasia is far more
generally accepted by ministers, priests, and rabbis than medical people
recognize or as yet even accept.) Humanist morality shows the same
nonabsolutistic attitude about preserving life. Indeed, not only Protestant, Catholic, and Jewish teaching take this stance; it is also true of
Buddhist, Hindu, and Moslem ethics. In short, the claim that we ought
always to do everything we can to preserve any patient's life as long as
possible is now discredited. The last serious advocate of this unconditional provitalist doctrine was David Karnofsky, the great tumor research scientist of the Sloan-Kettering Institute in New York. The issue
about *negative* (indirect) euthanasia is settled ethically.

Given modern medicine's capabilities, always to do what is technically
possible to prolong life would be morally indefensible on any ground
other than a vitalistic outlook. That is, the opinion that biological
survival is the first-order value and that all other considerations, such as
personality, dignity, well-being, and self-possession, necessarily take
second place. Vestigial last-ditch provitalists still mumble threateningly
about "what the Nazis did," but in fact the Nazis never engaged in
euthanasia or mercy killing. What they did was merciless killing, either
for genocidal or ruthless experimental purposes.

One way of putting this is to say that the traditional ethics based on the
sanctity of life, which was the classical doctrine of medical idealism in its
prescientific phases, must give way to an ethics of the *quality* of life. This
comes about for humane reasons. It is a result of modern medicine's
successes, not failures. "New occasions teach new duties, time makes
ancient good uncouth," as Whittier said.

There are many pre-ethical or metaethical issues that are often over-
looked in ethical discussions. People of equally good reasoning powers
and a high respect for the rules of inference will still puzzle and even
infuriate each other. This is because they fail to see that their moral judgments proceed from significantly different values, ideals, and starting
points. If God's will (perhaps "specially revealed" in the Bible or "generally revealed" in his Creation) is against any responsible human initiative in the dying process, or if sheer life is believed to be, as such, more
desirable than anything else, then those who hold these opinions will not
find much merit in any case we might make for either kind of euthanasia,
direct or indirect. If, on the other hand, the highest good is personal

integrity and human well-being, then euthanasia in either form could or might be the right thing, depending on the situation. This latter kind of ethics is the key to what will be said in this chapter.

Let's say it again, clearly, for the sake of truly serious ethical discourse. Many of us look upon living and dying as we do upon health and medical care, as person-centered. This is not a solely or basically biological understanding of what it means to be "alive" and to be "dead." It asserts that a so-called vegetable, the brain-damaged victim of an auto accident or a microcephalic newborn or a case of massive neurologic deficit and lost cerebral capacity, who nevertheless goes on breathing and whose midbrain or brain stem continues to support spontaneous organ functions, is in such a situation no longer a human being, no longer a person, no longer really alive. It is *personal* function that counts, not biological function. Humanness is understood as primarily rational, not physiological. This "doctrine of man" puts the *homo* and *ratio* before the *vita*. It holds that being human is more valuable than being alive.

All of this is said just to make it clear from the outset that biomedical progress is forcing us, whether we welcome it or not, to make fundamental *conceptual* changes as well as scientific and medical changes. Not only are the conditions of life and death changing, because of our greater control and, in consequence, our greater decision-making responsibility; our *definitions* of life and death also have to change to keep pace with the new realities.

These changes are signaled in a famous surgeon's remark recently: "When the brain is gone there is no point in keeping anything else going." What he meant was that with an end of cerebration, i.e., the function of the cerebral cortex, the *person* is gone (dead) no matter how many other spontaneous or artificially supported functions persist in the heart, lungs, and vascular system. Such noncerebral processes might as well be turned off, whether they are natural or artificial.

This conclusion is of great philosophical and religious interest because it reaffirms the ancient Christian-European belief that the core of humanness, of the *humanum*, lies in the *ratio*—man's rational faculty. It is not the loss of brain function in general but of cerebral function (the synthesizing "mind") in particular that establishes that death has ensued.

Using the old conventional conceptual apparatus, we naturally thought about both life and death as events, not as processes, which, of course, they are. We supposed that these events or episodes depended on the accidents of nature or in some kind of special providence. It is therefore no surprise to hear people grumbling that a lot of the decision making that has to be carried out in modern medical care is playing God. And given that way of thinking, the only possible answer to the charge is to accept it: Yes, we *are* playing God. But the real question is: Which or whose God are we playing?

In their growing up spiritually, men are now turning to a "God" who or which is the creative principle behind things—behind the test tube as much as behind the earthquake and volcano. This can be believed, but the old God's sacralistic inhibitions on human freedom and research can no longer be submitted to.

We must rid ourselves of that obsolete theodicy according to which God is not only the cause but also the builder of nature and its works, and not only the builder but even the manager. That archaic view made God himself the efficient as well as the final cause of earthquake and fire, of life and death, and by logical inference any interference with nature (which is exactly what medicine is) was impious. Ethically, it was unresponsible.

Most of our major moral problems are posed by scientific discoveries and by the subsequent technical know-how we gain, in the control of life and health and death. Ethical questions jump out at us from every laboratory and clinic. May we exercise these controls at all, we wonder—and if so, then when, where, how? Every advance in medical capabilities is an increase in our moral responsibility, a widening of the range of our decision-making obligations.

Genetics, molecular biology, fetology, and obstetrics have developed to a point where we now have effective control over the start of human life's continuum. From now on it would be irresponsible to leave baby making to mere chance and impulse, as we once *had* to do.

What has taken place in birth control is equally imperative in death control. The whole armory of resuscitation and prolongation of life forces us to be responsible decision makers about death as much as about birth; there must be quality control in the terminating of life as in its initiating. It is ridiculous to give ethical approval to the positive ending of subhuman life *in utero*, as we do in therapeutic abortions for reasons of mercy and compassion, but refuse to approve of positively ending a subhuman life *in extremis*. If we are morally obliged to put an end to a pregnancy when an amniocentesis reveals a terribly defective fetus, we are equally obliged to put an end to a patient's hopeless misery when a brain scan reveals that a patient with cancer has advanced brain metastases.

Only man is aware of death. Animals know pain, and fear it, but not death. Furthermore, in humans the ability to meet death and even to regard it sometimes as a friend is a sign of manliness. But in the new patterns of medicine and health care patients tend to die in a moribund or comatose state, so that death comes without the patient's knowledge.

The Elizabethan litany's petition, "...from sudden death, good Lord, deliver us," has become irrelevant much if not most of the time.

It is because of this incompetent condition of so many of the dying that we cannot discuss the ethical issues of elective death only in the narrow terms of voluntary, patient-chosen euthanasia. A careful typology of elective death will distinguish at least five forms—five ways of dying which are not willy-nilly blind chance but matters of choice, purpose, and responsible freedom. (Historical ethics and moral theology are obviously major sources of suggestion for these distinctions.)

1. *Active, voluntary, direct.* This is death chosen and carried out by the patient. The most familiar way is the overdose left near at hand for the patient. It is a matter of simple request and of personal liberty. In a word, it is suicide. In any particular case, we might properly raise the question of the patient's competence, but to hold that euthanasia in this category is justifiable entails a rejection of the simplistic canard that all suicides are mentally disordered.

Presumably a related issue arises around the conventional notion of consent in medical ethics. The codes (American Medical Association, Helsinki, World Medical Association, Nuremberg) all contend that valid consent to any surgery or treatment requires a reasonable prospect of benefit to the patient. What, then, is benefit? Could death in some situations be a benefit? As a question in the relativity of values, my own answer is in the affirmative.

2. *Passive, voluntary, direct.* The choice might be made either *in situ* or long in advance of a terminal illness, e.g., by exacting a promise that if and when Shakespeare's "bare bodkin" or potion cannot be self-administered, somebody will do it for the patient. In this case the patient gives to others—physicians, lawyers, family, friends—the discretion to end it all as and when the situation requires, if the patient becomes comatose or too dysfunctioned to take the necessary steps himself.

3. *Passive, voluntary, indirect.* This, like the second form, is done for, rather than by, the patient, but with his consent and by indirect means only, not directly. A directive or form called the Living Will is in wide use, with legal enforcement in some states (but not all). For example, in these right-to-die laws the recorded wish of a comatose or suffering patient (if, and only if, the patient is terminally ill) is protected from those who would disregard the patient's directive to have all treatment stopped. Hospital staff, physicians, and family often try to do this. As people learn to fear senescence more than death (a fear brought about by undiscriminating resuscitation practices), this policy spreads. Neither the common law tradition nor statute law is equipped to deal with the anti-euthanasia culture-lag. (In Italy, Germany, and Switzerland the law

provides for a reduction of penalties when it is done at the patient's request.)

4. *Passive, involuntary, direct.* This is the form or procedure in which a simple "mercy killing" is done on a patient's behalf without his present or prior consent. Instances would be when an idiot is given a fatal dose, or the death of a child in the worst stages of Tay-Sachs disease is speeded along, or when a man trapped inextricably in a blazing fire is shot to end his suffering, or a shutdown is ordered on a patient deep in a mindless condition, irreversibly, perhaps due to an injury or an infection or some biological breakdown. It is this form of euthanasia which has posed the problem several times in court trials and indictments.

To my knowledge, Uruguay is the only country that allows it. Article 37 of the *Codiga Penal* specifically states that although it is a "crime" *pro forma* the courts are authorized to forego any penalty. In time the world will follow suit. Laws in Colombia and in the Soviet Union (Article 50 of the Code of Criminal Procedure) are similar to Uruguay's, but in those codes freedom from punishment is allowed but not normative.

The conflict and tension between stubborn prohibitionism on the one hand and a humane compassion on the other may be seen in the legal history of the issue in the United States. Eleven cases of "mercy killing" have actually reached the courts: one was on a charge of voluntary manslaughter, with a conviction and penalty of three to six years in prison and a $500 fine; one was for first-degree murder, resulting in a conviction which was promptly reduced to a penalty of six years in jail with immediate parole. All of the other nine cases were twisted into "temporary insanity" or no-proof judgments. In short, no convictions.

5. Finally, *passive, involuntary, indirect.* This is the "letting the patient go" tactic which is being acted out every day in our hospitals. Nothing is done for the patient positively to release him from his tragic condition (other than "trying to make him comfortable"). What is done is done *for* him rather than in response to any request by him. It is an uninstructed proxy decision. As we all know, even this passive policy of compassion is followed only grudgingly, much of the time. It continues to be at least theoretically vulnerable to malpractice and criminal-neglect suits under the lagging law—brought, possibly, by angry or venal members of the family or litigious lawyers.

Ethically regarded, however, this euthanasia practice is manifestly superficial, morally timid, and evasive of the real issue. I repeat: it is harder morally to justify letting somebody die a slow and ugly death, dehumanized, than it is to justify helping him to avoid it.

What, then, is the real issue? In a few words, it is whether we can morally justify taking it into our own hands, as human beings, to hasten death for ourselves (suicide) or for others (mercy killing) out of reasons of compassion. The answer in my view is clearly yes, on both sides of it. Indeed, *to justify either one, suicide or mercy killing, is to justify the other.*

The heart of the matter analytically is the question of whether the end justifies the means. If the end sought is the patient's death as a release from pointless misery and dehumanization, then the requisite or appropriate means is justified. The old maxim of some moral theologians was *finis sanctificat media.* The point is that no act is anything but random and *meaningless* unless it is purposefully related to some end or object. To be moral an act must be seeking an end. However, to hold that the end justifies the means does not entail the absurd notion that *any* means can be justified by *any* end. The priority of the end is paired with the principle of 'proportionate good'; any dysvalue in the means must be outweighed by the value gained in the end. In systems analysis, with its pragmatic approach, the language would be: the benefit must repay the cost or the trade-off is not justified. It comes down to this, that in some situations a morally good end can justify a relatively bad means, on the principle of proportionate good.

The really searching question of conscience is, therefore, whether we are right in believing that *the well-being of persons* is the highest good. If so, then it follows that either suicide or mercy killing could be the right thing to do in some exigent and tragic circumstances. This could be the case, for instance, when an incorrigible human vegetable, whether spontaneously functioning or artificially supported, is progressively degraded while constantly eating up private or public financial resources in violation of the distributive justice owed to others. In such cases the patient is actually already departed and only his body is left, and the needs of others have a stronger claim upon us morally. The fair allocation of scarce resources is as profound an ethical obligation as any we can imagine in a civilized society, and it arises very practically at the clinical level when triage officers make their decisions at the expense of some patients' needs in favor of others'.

Another way of putting this is to say that the crucial question is not whether the end justifies the means (what else could?) but *what justifies the end?* And this chapter's answer is, plainly and confidently, that human happiness and well-being is the highest good or *summum bonum,* and that therefore any ends or purposes which that standard or ideal validates are just, right, good. This is what humanistic medicine is all about; it is what the concepts of loving concern and social justice are built upon.

This position comes down to the belief that our moral acts, including suicide and mercy killing, are right or wrong depending on the consequences aimed at (we sometimes fail, of course, through ignorance or poor reasoning), and that the consequences are good or evil according to whether and how much they serve human values. This is precisely a "consequential" moral judgment.

I believe that this mode of ethics is both implicit and explicit in the morality of medical care and biomedical research. Its reasoning is inductive, not deductive, and it proceeds empirically from the data of each actual case or problem, choosing the course that offers an optimum or maximum of desirable consequences. Medicine is not *a prioristic* or *prejudiced* in its ethos and modalities, and therefore to proscribe either suicide or mercy killing is so blatantly nonconsequential that it calls for critical scrutiny. It fails to make sense. It is unclinical and doctrinaire.

The problem exists because of the other kind of ethics which holds that we ought or ought not to do certain things no matter how good or bad the consequences might foreseeably be. Such rules are prohibitions or taboos, expressed as thou-shalt-nots. While my ethics is teleological or end-oriented, the opposite approach is *deontological* (from the Greek *deonteis*, meaning duty); i.e., it is duty-ethics, not goal-ethics. Its advocates sometimes sneer at any determination of obligation in terms of consequences, calling it "a mere morality of goals."

In duty-ethics what is right is whatever act obeys or adheres to the rules, even though the foreseeable result will be inhumane. That is, its highest good is not human happiness and well-being but obedience to a rule—or what we might call a prejudiced or predetermined decision based not on the clinical variables but on some transcending "principle."

For example, the fifth of the Ten Commandments, which prohibits killing, is cited as a strict prohibition for nonconsequentialists when it comes to killing in the service of humane values like mercy and compassion, and yet at the same time they ignore their "moral law" when it comes to self-defense. The egocentricity and solipsism in this moral posture, which is a very common one, never ceases to bemuse consequentialists. You may end your neighbor's life for your own sake, but you may not do it for his sake! And you may end your own life for your neighbor's sake, as in an act of sacrificial heroism, but you may not end your life for your own sake. This is a veritable mare's nest of nonsense!

The plain hard logic of it is that the end or purpose of both negative and positive euthanasia is exactly the same: to contrive or bring about the patient's death. Acts of deliberate omission are morally not different from acts of commission. But in the Anglo-American *law*, it is a crime to push a blind man off a cliff. It is not, however, a crime to deliberately not lift a finger to prevent his walking over the edge. This is an unpleasant feature of legal reasoning which is alien to ethics and to a sensitive conscience. Ashamed of it, even the courts fall back on such legal fictions as insanity in euthanasia cases, and this has the predictable effect of undermining our respect for the law.

There is something obviously evasive when we rule motive out in charging people with the crime of mercy killing, but then bring it back in again for purposes of determining punishment! It is also a menacing delimitation of the concepts of culpability, responsibility, and negligence. No *ethically* disciplined decision maker could so blandly separate right and wrong from motives, foresight, and consequences. (Be it noted, however, that motive is taken into account in German and Swiss law, and that several European countries provide for recognition of "homicide when requested" as a special category.)

It is naive and superficial to suppose that because we don't do anything positively to hasten a patient's death we have thereby avoided complicity in his death. Not doing anything is doing something; it is a decision to act every bit as much as deciding for any other deed. If I decide not to eat or drink any more, knowing what the consequence will be, I have committed suicide as surely as if I had used a gas oven. If physicians decide not to open an imperforate anus in a severe 21-trisomy newborn, they have committed mercy killing as surely as if they had used a poison pellet!

Let the reader at this point now ask himself once more if he is a consequentialist or an *a priori* decision maker; and again, let him ask himself if he is a humanist or alternatively has something he holds to be better than the well-being of human beings. (Thoughtless religious people will sometimes point out that we are required to love God as well as our neighbors, but can the two loves ever come into conflict? Actually, is there any way to love God other than through the neighbor? Only mystics imagine that they can love God directly and discretely.)

Occasionally I hear a physician say that he could not bring himself to resort to direct euthanasia. That may be so. What anybody would do in such tragic situations is a problem in psychology, however, not in ethics. We are not asking what we would do but what we *should* do. Any of us who has an intimate knowledge of what happens in terminal illnesses can tell stories of rational people—both physicians and family—who were quite clear ethically about the rightness of an overdose or of "turning off the machine," and yet found themselves too inhibited to give the word or do the deed. That is a phenomenon of primary interest to psychology, and of only incidental interest to ethics.

Careful study of the best texts of the Hippocratic Oath shows that it says nothing at all about preserving life, as such. It says that "so far as power and discernment shall be mine, I will carry out regimen for the benefit of the sick and will keep them from harm and wrong." The case for euthanasia depends upon how we understand "benefit of the sick" and "harm" and "wrong." If we regard dehumanized and merely bio-logical life as sometimes real harm and the very opposite of benefit, to refuse to welcome or even introduce death would be quite wrong mor-ally.

In most states in this country people now can, and do, carry cards, legally enforceable, which explain the carrier's wish that when he dies his organs and tissue should be used for transplant when needed by the living. The day will come when people will also be able to carry a card, notarized and legally executed, which explains that they do not want to be kept alive beyond the *humanum* point, and authorizing the ending of their biological processes by any of the methods of euthanasia which seems appropriate. In the year 1977 alone, eight states in the United States adopted Right-to-Die laws, providing for what I have called in-direct and involuntary euthanasia, but the other forms will one day be socially accepted and enacted into law. Suicide may or may not be the ultimate problem of philosophy, as Albert Camus thought it is, but in any case it is the ultimate problem of medical ethics.

Thirteen

Cerebration

Starting in the first chapter of this volume there has been a kind of refrain to the effect that a genuinely human being is able to think, at whatever level the qualifying minimum is set. We ought to regard the *ratio* and not the *vita* as the key to the *homo*. The following historical-philosophical footnote is worth some thought.

In 1968, a man named Bruce Tucker, unconscious from massive head injuries, was wheeled into the Medical College of Virginia in Richmond very late one night. The next day he was pronounced dead. After a vigorous, unsuccessful police search for his family (his body was not claimed) the doctors at MCV made him an involuntary donor in a heart transplant operation. Under the Unclaimed Bodies Act, they were allowed to transplant his heart into the chest of a patient dying of cardiac failure. Despite the operation, the recipient, Joseph Klett, died a week later.

Though this incident was obscure at the time, it was to spark a landmark legal decision concerning the definition of death. This definition is of surpassing importance to the medical profession and to society because of medicine's astonishing advances in life-support technology.

The case in point first became public in 1972 in a celebrated trial in the Richmond Law and Equity Court and came to be known as the Richmond Brain Case, or the Tucker Trial. The case was built on a charge of wrongful death brought by William Tucker, a brother who had finally been located, against the hospital and the fourteen physicians involved in the transplant. To sharpen the contest, a hundred thousand dollars damages were demanded as reparation.

First a look at the trial, and then we can focus on its outcome, with special reference to the medical and moral issues involved. Other cases of this nature have occurred, but the Tucker trial set a precedent in defining when death takes place.

Since I played a part in the trial, I should explain how I became involved. Four months earlier, in January, the Virginia Bar Association listened to a panel discussion about the cultural lag between existing law, both common and statute, concerning the determination of death and the application of the law. This lag had been caused largely by the rapid introduction of modern medical techniques.

The panel's chairman was Walter Wadlington, James Madison Professor of Law at the University of Virginia, who was paired with Richard Williams, a distinguished trial lawyer. Medicine was represented by Thomas Hunter, M.D., Owen Cheatham Professor of Science at the university. As Visiting Professor of Medical Ethics at the University, I completed the foursome.

Having heard the panel, and with its revelations fresh in mind, the chief defense counsel for the physicians, Mr. Jack Russell, called me as soon as a date was set for the trial. He asked if I would testify as a non-medical expert witness about the philosophical and theological aspects of determining death. In effect, I was to explain the case for viewing death as the end of personal identity, rather than as the end of breathing and heartbeat.

Judge Christian Compton at first took the common-sense line that the court's business was to interpret and apply the law, not to make it, that the Virginia law on determining death agreed with *Black's Legal Dictionary*: "...death...is defined as...a total stoppage of the circulation of the blood, and a cessation of the animal and vital functions consequent thereto such as respiration and pulsation."

Therefore, he held that if medical opinion has swung in favor of a neurological definition, i.e., brain or coma death, this new position should be a question for the state legislature, not the courts.

Judge Compton further held that charges against the transplant team must be dropped, because the surgeons had acted after the determination of Tucker's death had been made by others. This gave what might be called "criminal relief" to the surgeons, David M. Hume, M.D. (who died a year after the trial in the crash of his private plane), Richard R. Lower, M.D., and David H. Sewall, M.D. But they were still professionally concerned, as everybody else was, about the medical problem of what constituted "reasonable efforts to prolong life" and how to understand when in fact death occurs.

The most seriously threatened physician among those indicted was Abdullah Fatteh, M.D., for he had made the determination of death and had given the surgeons consent to remove Bruce Tucker's heart. The plaintiff contended that Dr. Fatteh's decision was erroneous. Bruce Tucker, they argued, was still alive at the time of the operation, for he still had a heartbeat, respiration, blood pressure and body temperature.

The first important turn of events during the trial occurred when Judge Compton reversed himself, in a sense, by broadening the trial's definition of death to include the medical or neurological definition as well as the statutory one. He was thereby allowing the jury to hear medical arguments concerning when death occurs. This testimony was provided by William Sweet, M.D., chief of neurosurgery at Massachusetts General Hospital, and William Collins, M.D., the eminent Yale neurosurgeon.

State Senator Douglas Wilder, Tucker's lawyer, mounted a long and earnest argument to prevent me from testifying, on the ground that my testimony would be neither factual as to what happened nor professionally medical. But in the end, I was allowed to testify as a "relevantly competent witness."

The defense attorney's first question to me was whether modern medicine has made the issue of understanding life and death more complicated. I replied, "If anything, modern neurological science has simplified it, given it more reliability. We no longer need refer to pulsation and other vital signs; we can go directly to the center of vitality itself, the brain."

Pressed by lawyers on both sides, I tried to state the problem simply: "The essence of the question lies in cerebral function. When that is gone, nothing remains but biological phenomena at best. The patient is gone even if his body remains, and even if some of its vital functions continue."

I was considered to be qualified because, if death is to be redefined as loss of certain brain functions, there are surely grave questions of theology and philosophy at stake. Hence, allowing me to take the stand was the second critical development.

There was another question in the case that threatened to override the medical and ethical issues, at least in the public's mind, and that was the issue of race. The plaintiff's attorney, Douglas Wilder, was the only black member of the Virginia Senate; the donor patient, the late Bruce Tucker, was black, while the recipient was white; and, finally, one of the jurors was black. But the racial red herring died in shallow water, in part because the attorney for the plaintiff creditably played down the race factor.

The seven-member (all male) jury took less than fifty minutes to find in the physicians' favor. They judged that the patient, Bruce Tucker, had died when his brain ceased to function, as the defense contended, and not when the surgeon removed his heart, as the plaintiff had argued.

As one juryman put it to a reporter for the *Richmond Times-Dispatch*, "It was clearly proved in the trial that a man...cannot live without a functioning brain." Another explained that the jury was convinced that "the existing legal definition of when death occurs is no longer acceptable."

So much for the case itself. What is its overriding meaning? The jury's decision was the first of its kind, but it certainly was not the last, and it raised probing questions about the meaning of such words as "human" and "alive" and "brain" and "death." Resuscitative medicine, life-support systems, neurology and brain physiology, along with transplant surgery with its pressures of timing, have forced us to take a long, hard, fresh look at these too familiar, unexamined terms and concepts.

To find answers, however, we may be forced to do more than just rearrange our mental furniture; we may have to scrap some of our conventional wisdom and instill a different conceptual apparatus altogether. For we have now reached a level of medical capability where we find ourselves unsure about the point at which we cross the line from extending life to prolonging death. Might it be that a patient is sometimes "alive" but no longer "human"?

If there are times when plugs should be pulled to let the patient die or when death may be pronounced even though vital functions, as distinguished from truly human functions, still operate, then we are going to have to face up to certain uncomfortable questions—questions that we find we have not by any means settled for all time. Can we, for example, go on speaking intelligently of "human vegetables" if the two terms are mutually exclusive? We are facing a big and very important package of questions concerning when, how, and why we may exercise any initiative and responsibility in death and dying.

But these related questions do not get at the central issue dramatized by the Richmond Brain Case. Stop and look again at the jurymen's posttrial remarks we have quoted. They tied their decision to something they had heard in the courtroom called "brain death," which, I submit, was and is the core issue. Is the death of the brain, as such, really what determines when death has occurred? I think a strong case can be made for holding that is not the proper definition.

There are few people today who would say that we should keep a person alive biologically as long as possible, even after he is lost as a person or has lost his capability for a personal existence. Sometimes, undiscriminating, over-zealous activists in intensive care units ignore the ethics of compassion when, for example, they resuscitate some cases of severe anoxia; many in medicine call this the ICU psychosis. There are, of course, a few vitalists for whom life itself is the highest good, but most of us are humanists for whom integrity and well-being are the highest good. Quality of life counts, not just quantity.

But even so, "brain death" is not the proper label for a realistic definition of death. Brain death is so broad in its language that it represents no real change from the old definition of death. That is, if the whole brain, including the brain stem and midbrain, as well as the cerebrum, must lose its functions to meet this definition, then obviously the whole neurologic system shuts down. In other words, the death of the entire brain is no different from the systemic death of traditional clinical determinations.

It is precisely upon this reasoning that the Harvard definition of death as coma will founder. Incidentally, this is also why it is uncritical to speak of the possibility someday of "brain transplants." Bodies are appendages of brains, not vice versa. The brain would always be the recipient; it would take over the grafted body and operate it with the brain's own stored knowledge.

When, then, should a person be considered dead? The death of the individual is the irreversible loss of whatever component in his biological system holds the essence of the person, and that component is the cerebrum in the brain, not the whole brain. This is the crucial point. What makes me or you is our cerebrum bilaterally—the cortex, white matter, basal ganglia, thalamus; this is where the sum of our experience, our personal history, is stored.

If we can affirm that in our value system personal existence or self-consciousness counts for more than the physical body, no matter how many other spontaneous functions may persist, because they are maintained by the noncortical brain (a "vegetable"), then *cerebral death* is the correct concept.

Paul MacLean of the National Institutes of Health has distinguished the three parts of the brain as they are separated by evolution and function: first, the reptilian or brain stem, the neurologic role of which is to deal with autonomic functions; second, the mammalian or midbrain, the so-called limbic system in which emotional controls are centered; and third, the human, or "new" brain, which *Homo sapiens* has developed in the past one million years.

The last part, the cerebral cortex, is what distinguishes men from subhuman animals. (Arthur Koestler and John Smythies make much of this, perhaps too much, in *Beyond Reductionism*.) The distinctive or peculiar trait of human beings is their mental power, the *ratio* that only they possess.

The cerebral cortex is where the "mind" is located. It is thought, cerebration, that makes us human, not simply the undifferentiated brain. Smart people are not brainy, if we use language precisely; they are cortexy or frontal-lobey. Thus, any serious attempt to explain what it means to be human, to define humanhood, inevitably runs into the problem of minimum IQ. Humanoid status calls for at least a thousand grams of brains, but human status calls for several billion neurons properly hooked up for storage, retrieval, and synthesis. The key is the cortex, or switchboard.

My purpose here is only to understand the real question posed by the Richmond Brain Case, the central or cardinal question on which every thing else hinges. Besides I.Q. or cerebral capacity, there are other precious indicators of humanhood.

Robert Sinsheimer of the California Institute of Technology, in *Genetic Engineering and Science*, has listed, besides self-awareness, perception of the past, present and future; the capacity for hope, love, and trust; an ability to communicate and participate, and to understand nature rationally; and a drive to reduce fate's role, along with a vision of man as unfinished.

But the heart of the matter, to use a phrase dear to Graham Greene, is that it is cerebral or mental function that is the key to authentically human life—and therefore the key to human death—and not the visceral sector, important as that is in the total range of human life. The cerebral function is the instrument of all the virtues or qualities we usually assign to truly human beings. Indeed, without cerebration, the limbic functions become inordinate and destructive.

I suppose it comes down to this: The human brain is clearly distinguished from the animal brain only by the frontal granular cortex.

When the cortex has not yet functioned or when it has finally ceased to function, there is no human life; human life has not started in the first case (fetal growth) and has ended in the other case (terminal or "vegetable" life.) Such are the problems the Richmond Brain Case opened up to the public record. It is a Pandora's box containing no less a riddle than the question, What qualities constitute humanhood?—a question most of us have long thought was answered by law and by custom.

I am still firmly of the opinion that the notion of whole-brain death is too broad. It is too broad because, if no part of the brain is functioning, then the traditional clinical criteria in Black's definition are necessarily also satisfied. It means that there is no real change in the law after all. On this basis, brain death and biological death are equivalent; total brain death is total death. Everything stops.

If we mean cerebral death, the loss of cerebral or cortical function, we should say so. The irreversible loss of cerebral function, of "thinking," may be what the *ad hoc* committee of Harvard's medical school wanted to establish, but if so, their criteria are so applied usually that "irreversible coma" means the patient is unable to maintain bodily functions spontaneously, i.e., without artificial support systems.

When, in another famous case, the parents of Karen Ann Quinlan asked the courts to let the machines be turned off, it was not in order to let her die but to see whether she would die "naturally" if left without an artificial support system. When the machines were disconnected, she proved to be in irreversible coma, a persistent vegetative state. Her brain still functioned in the part that regulates autonomic functions (breathing, blood pressure, heart rate); only the cognitive brain function, cerebration, was gone.

New Jersey's Supreme Court found in favor of turning off the machines, on the assumption that Karen could no longer breathe on her own. They were turned off and she still went on "living." How long she could "live" this way nobody knows. The brain stem or reptilian brain keeps her going. However, if her loss of cerebral function meant that she, the person Karen, was dead, then we face what I take to be the real issue. Can the excerebral, decorticate patient, with no thinking brain, be held to be dead even though the body lives? The real ethical question for medicine and survivors has walked out on the stage. When cerebral death has occurred, why not stop the care as well as the treatment? Code Nine labels usually mean, "Care, no treatment." In situations such as these, is intravenous feeding treatment? or care? What is the difference? What is the point? This is what we are left to wonder.

Fourteen

Suicide

Choosing a "good death," which is a literal translation of *euthanasia*, is usually thought to be justifiable when death is near at hand, in terminal illness. But to choose death quite apart from natural causes is different; we call it suicide. As one form of elective death, it invites a closer scrutiny.

John Donne, poet and dean of St. Paul's, when his friend Ben Jonson was ruling the London literary roost in Tudor-Stuart times, wrote a tough-minded essay on ethics: *Biothanatos: A Declaration of that Paradoxe, or Thesis, That Self-homicide is not so naturally Sinne, that it may never be otherwise* (1611).

Later, however, becoming an eminent divine in the Establishment, Donne repudiated his own thesis. Having no prospect nor desire to be dean of St. Paul's, I can promise the reader that I will make no such turnaround, to deny what this essay says. Donne also theologized the question when he declared that Jesus had committed suicide in order to bring about mankind's salvation. Again unlike the poet-preacher, I promise not to engage here in any flights of soteriology, no cosmic hypotheses of ultimate euphoria.

Anthropologists have found every imaginable attitude toward suicide in both savage and civilized societies. However, like psychiatrists and sociologists, they are able only to provide us with data. In their scientific capacity they cannot jump the gap between what is and what ought to be. To suppose that we can settle an ethical question by tabulating moral sentiments, discovered through observation, is the 'naturalistic' fallacy—confusing what is with what ought to be. Whether we ought to be free to end our lives or not is a question of philosophy, of ethics in particular. If a psychiatrist, for example, asserts or implies that people ought not to choose naughtness or oblivionate themselves (Herman Melville's neologisms), he is wearing his philosopher's hat. "Ought" is not in the scientific lexicon.

In spite of the defiant immortalists who look forward to resurrection by cryonics or by outwitting cell death biochemically (Alan Harrington: "Death is an imposition on the human race, and no longer acceptable"), we know perfectly well that aging is a fatal disease, and all of us are its victims. The ethical question is whether we may ever rightly take the initiative in death and dying or are, instead, obliged in conscience to look upon life and death fatalistically, as something which has to just *happen* to us willy-nilly.

We have pretty well settled the life control issue with our contraceptive practices and policies. Now we have to look just as hard at the death control problem. If we may initiate life, may we not terminate it? Were Ernest Hemingway, and his father before him, wrong to shoot themselves? Ethically? Psychologically?

From the vantage point of moral philosophy, the main thing is to posit at the outset that no action is intrinsically right or wrong, nothing is inherently good or evil. Right and wrong, good and evil, desirable and undesirable—all are ethical terms, and all are predicates. Not properties. Values and the morality of human acts are contingent, depending on the shape of the action in the situation, *Sitz im Leben* or *Situationsethik*. The variables and factors in each set of circumstances are the determinants of what ought to be done.

There simply is no way to prove or defend our values by logic; they are established for us or in us by a mixture of conditioning, choice, and commitment. Recall Ludwig Wittgenstein's confession: "This is a terrible business—just terrible. You can at best stammer when you talk of it."

On the other hand, when it comes to acting as a moral agent, tailoring our deeds to fit our values and ideals, we have to use logic and critical reason, especially when we have to decide which values get priority when they compete for our preference. If truthtelling, for example, has a high-order value but it conflicts with a therapeutic goal, telling the truth might sometimes be the *wrong* thing to do.

To suppose that we would always be obliged to follow any rule of conduct is only tenable on a metaphysical basis or because of an alleged revelation of eternal absolutes. Such universals are what the Greeks called the *proton pseudon*, the basic error, of conventional (i.e., unexamined) moralism. Most Christian and many Jewish moralists use starting points of this kind. Without such supernatural buttressing, however, any attempt to assign intrinsic moral value to anything—truth, chastity, property, health, or even life itself—is an abysmal ethical mistake.

Stepping for a moment into another context, the point at stake can be brought home by quoting a question-and-answer column in a religious magazine: "*Q*. My wife is sterile but wants her 'marital rights.' I have a contagious venereal disease. May I wear a prophylactic sheath? *A*. No. Even though she could not conceive and you would infect her, contraceptive intercourse is an intrinsically evil act." Here it is in a nutshell. The situation makes no difference. The end sought makes no difference. The consequences make no difference. Nothing makes any difference. The act itself is wrong. This is the essence of "intrinsic" morality.

The typical moral theologian would condemn a captured soldier's heroic suicide to avoid betraying his comrades under torture—because suicide is held to be an evil thing-in-itself, like Kant's *Ding-an-sich*, a defiance of the will of God. Against that kind of dogmatic sanction, an empirical or clinical ethics would have to agree that suicide can be right sometimes, wrong sometimes.

A slight variant on saying "suicide is not right" is to say "we have no right" to end our lives by choice. People are always mixing human "rights" and right conduct together. Thoughtless talk about rights is a form of the same legalistic *a priori* or predetermined moral judgment that we hear when people say "it isn't right"—whether the "it" is suicide or breaking a promise or committing adultery or stealing something, or any other act.

In humanistic ethics, when suicide helps human beings it is right. That is, we have a "right" to do it. What makes it right is human need. Human rights, as I have contended, are not self-validating; they are not intrinsically valid. It is need that validates rights, not the other way around. When rights are asserted over against or cutting across human needs, we are faced with a set of superhuman or supernatural moral principles; they are often in practice callous and cruel contradictions of a humane morality.

Donne's contemporary, William Shakespeare, puts the ethical question this way: "Then is it sin,/To rush into the secret home of death,/Ere death dare come to us?" Cassio, though a good Catholic, thought Othello's suicide was noble. The priest did not condemn the self-conclusion chosen by Romeo and Juliet. Even though Ophelia was censured by the ecclesiastics, Shakespeare himself never expressed the kind of moralistic horror we find in Dante, who put suicides in the Seventh Circle of hell (lower than murderers and heretics). As a matter of fact, few cultures or traditions have ever condemned suicide out of whole cloth, indiscriminately.

The story of what various people have thought and done about suicide does not, *eo ipso*, settle the problem of what is right and good about it. Yet even so, the pages of history tell us things that help us to put the ethics of elective death in perspective. We might just look at the record in capsule.

Europe, Asia, Africa, America, all tell much the same story. Suicide is seen as absurd and tragic, noble and mean, brave and cowardly, sane and silly; every way of judging it has been taken. Some of the religious and superstitious have condemned it wholesale, others have even praised it. For example, the Koran held that suicide interfered with *kismet*, Allah's control of human life and destiny, making it as much as or more to be condemned than homicide. Cardinal Richelieu professed the same opinion. Other religions, on the other hand, have honored suicides. This was the case among the American Indians, upon whom genocide was inflicted by the Christian conquistadores Cortez and Pizarro, whose Spanish priests were at the same time condemning the Indians' selective suicide. Other examples of religious suicide would be the Japanese rite of *seppuku* or *hara-kiri*, and the Brahmans' *suttee*. Monkish protests against Thieu's dictatorship in South Vietnam by self-immolation were comparable.

The Buddhist admiration for *banzai* and *kamikaze* is more complicated ethically, because suicidal practices of that order combine killing oneself with killing others. Something like *banzai* is to be seen in the suicidal commando tactics of Palestinian guerillas, and in the "living bomb" gestures of Viet Cong terrorists. The supposed difference between the suicidal practice of *banzai* and volunteering to fly in the Luftwaffe bombers, or as RAF pilots in the Battle of Britain, poses an interesting analytic problem (speaking ethically, not psychiatrically).

More primitive peoples often believed that a suicide's soul or ghost would wander around without a resting place, haunting the living. To prevent this in medieval Christendom, they buried them with a stake through the heart, digging the grave at a crossroads instead of in "hallowed" (blessed) ground, to keep it from poisoning the soil. The Baganda people followed a similar defense strategy, as the famed missionary Livingston found when he stayed among them. The Alabama Indians threw their suicides' bodies into the river; in Dahomey, they threw them to carrion. But as often as culture groups made suicide taboo, others affirmed or even revered it. In North America the Zuni frowned on it, but the Navajo and Hopi did not; in the Pacific it was condemned in the Andaman Islands, praised in the Fijis.

The Bible never condemned suicide, although in later times the rabbinical Talmud did and the Christian church followed suit. Samson, Saul, Abimilech, Achitophel—their stories are told without censure. It was not until the sixth century that the act was proscribed in Europe. Until that time, in the absence of biblical authority, its condemnation had to be inferred from the sixth of the Ten Commandments, "Thou shalt not kill." The term "suicide" itself does not appear until the seventeenth century.

The Greeks, being more judicious, were therefore more selectively pro-suicide than the Jews, and so were the Romans. Both Stoics and Epicureans approve it in principle. Zeno approved, and so did Cleanthes. Seneca actually carried it out, to forestall the murderous Nero's fun and games, and Seneca's wife Paulina attempted to join him in it, but was thwarted by Nero's order. On the other hand, the Pythagoreans, opponents of Hippocratic medicine, claiming to have a special knowledge of the gods' decrees, opposed suicide because of what Islam later called *kismet*. (After all, if you "know" what a transcendental and ultimate will forbids, it makes a certain kind of prudential sense not to do it, *nicht wahr?*)

Plato allowed euthanasia, as Aristotle did, directly as suicide, not just as a matter of "letting the patient go." Homer and Euripides thought well of Jocasta's suicide after she learned that her new husband Oedipus was her own son—which was, perhaps, an excessive and irrational reaction, but humanly understandable, given the strength of the incest taboo. The Romans, as we all know, allowed the *liber mori* for a great many reasons. They denied it only to criminals, soldiers, and slaves, for obvious military and economic reasons. Justinian's *Digest* spelled the whole thing out to leave no doubt.

Christian Europe started moving away from pagan Rome's compassionate regard for the dignity of free persons, to the savagery of an undiscriminating condemnation of all suicide in the Middle Ages after the Graeco-Roman civilization had been ended by the Barbarian-Teutonic hordes. Once the classical philosophy was buried, the Catholic-medieval synthesis took over, and one of its first major elements was an absolute taboo on suicide. In the manorial system nearly everybody was enfeoffed to somebody else; hence suicide was, in effect, a soldier's or a slave's unlawful escape from somebody's possession. Suicide was fundamentally subversive of property rights.

They never put it that plainly, of course. Instead, they said that human life is a divine monopoly. "Our lives are God's." To take one's own life, therefore, is to invade Jesus Christ's property rights, for he had saved us "and we are therefore his." This mystical theology was the bottom layer of the moral and canonical prohibition. It led some of them to say that Judas Iscariot's suicide in remorse and despair was more wicked even than his earlier betrayal of Jesus and the consequent crucifixion.

A FALSE TURNING POINT

St. Augustine was the turning point in the hardening process. He was the first to absolutize the prohibition. None of the later antisuicide moralists improved on him; even Aquinas added only, "It is unnatural," thus reinforcing the theological ban with a religious metaphysics of natural law. An outline of Augustine's objections to suicide includes four propositions:

(1) If we are innocent, we may not kill the innocent; and if we are guilty, we may not take justice into our own hands. (2) The sixth commandment of the Decalogue forbids it, *non occides*; suicide is homicide, a felony, *felo de se*. (3) Our duty is to bear suffering with fortitude; not to is to duck out of our role as soldiers of Christ. (4) Suicide is the worst sin because it precludes repentance; to commit it in a state of grace after you are saved (cleansed of sin by Christ's blood) means you die out of grace (unsaved, eternally lost or damned). He allowed an occasional exception, however, for martyrs who had God's express directive or "guidance" to kill themselves. In such cases they were acting as innocently as those who sin *ex ignorantia inculpata* (in "invincible" ignorance). This is the argument Augustine used to answer the Donatists, a Christian sect which pointed out, reasonably enough, that dying baptized in a state of grace, by your own hand, was better than living long enough to fall back into sin, thus losing your chance to have eternal life in heaven.

At the end of the Holy Roman hegemony people began to reason again. By 1516 Thomas More (the "man for all seasons" who died for conscience's sake) had allowed suicide in his *Utopia*, even though Sir Thomas Browne frowned on it in his *Religio Medici* (1642). Montaigne backed More. And so it went. The great classic coup de grâce to the moral prohibition of suicide came with David Hume's essay "On Suicide" (1777), in which he reasoned that if it is wrong it must be because it offends God, or one's neighbor, or one's self, and then showed how this would not always be true on any of the three scores. He was joined by Voltaire, Rousseau, Montesquieu, d'Halbach.

The conventional wisdom persisted unchanged; attempted suicides were still hanged from the public gibbet. In Christian France, as in animist Dahomey, they threw the bodies on the garbage dump. The property of suicides was confiscated in England until 1870, and prison was the legal penalty for attempts until 1961. For the last hundred years or more the law has been evaded by the courts, because of their moral inhibition and ambivalence about suicide. They made a distinction between "suicide while of unsound mind" (legal "insanity") and *felo de se*, a punishable offense—the latter seldom if ever being the judgment actually reached. To echo C. E. M. Joad's observation, if you failed at suicide you were a criminal, and if you succeeded you were a lunatic. Hence the remarkable silence of ethical or legal literature on the subject.

At last, in the Suicide Act of 1961, England stopped making it a crime for a person, whether well or ill, to end his life or attempt to. There are only a few places left in the world where the courts still have to catch up with moral "sanity." Courts of law nowadays are seldom as unethical about suicide as the conventional moralists continue to be.

Always and everywhere we find cultural variety and difference along the spectrum of ethical opinion, running from blanket prohibition to selective justification. In a very sane and discrimiating fashion most communities, both savage and civilized, have believed that disposing of one's own life is like disposing of one's own property, a personal election. Except, of course, that in both life and property justice might forbid it if innocent third parties are victimized or the community suffers unfairly.

It was really on this last ground that most governments in the West opposed suicide. They followed Aristotle and Plato, who contended pragmatically that, except for *grave* reasons, suicide seriously deprives the community of soldiers needed to defend it and workers needed to do its labor of head and hand. This objection now, in an age of overpopulation, cybernated warfare, and automated industry, has little or no weight. The "right' to die is not right if and when it invades the well-being of others, but on the other hand, when it is truly a private choice it *is* right. To deny this is to deny the integrity of persons, to reduce them to mere functions or appendages of church and state.

Just as facts cannot tell us which things to value (although they help) nor how to rank them in a priorities order, neither can typologies. This caution applies, for example, to Emile Durkheim's famous classification of suicides into egoistic and altruistic, which is close to what we have come to mean in more recent days by "inner directed" and "other directed"—using the language of Riesman's *Lonely Crowd*.

Strong self-sustaining personalities are able (have the "ego strength") to defy cultural disapproval when or if a balance of pro-life and pro-death factors seem to weigh against going on living. As Albert Camus said, "Judging whether life is or is not worth living amounts to answering the fundamental question of philosophy."

On the "altruistic" side, there are times when sacrificial love and loyalty may call on us for a tragic decision, to choose death for the sake of a wider good than self. The decision is made pragmatically, as the greater good or the lesser evil. One thinks of Captain Oates in the Antarctic, who eliminated himself to speed up the escape of his companions, or of dysfunctioned grandparents pushing off on ice floes to relieve hungry Eskimos, or of the brave men who stayed on the sinking Titanic or dropped off from overloaded lifeboats.

Durkheim had a third type of suicides, the "anomic"—those who suffer *anomie*, who despair either for subjective reasons (including psychogenic illness) or objective reasons (maybe unemployability or social rejection). They reach a point where they "couldn't care less." Demoralized, unnerved, disoriented, they throw in their remaining chips. Suicides of *anomie*, like those done out of ego strength or for loyalty reasons, may or may not be rationally well-founded and prudent. Suicides of all kinds, in any typology, can be wise, or they can be foolish.

This is perhaps the point at which to challenge directly and flatly the widespread assumption that suicides are sick people, out of their minds. This canard has lodged itself very deeply even in the mental attitudes of physicians. It has managed to become the conventional wisdom of psychiatric medicine—partly, no doubt, because psychiatrists deal so much with false suicides whose verbal or nonverbal threats or "attempts" are signals of emotional or mental distress. Nevertheless, the idea is basically silly.

Like universalized or absolutized moral norms, this is undiscriminating; it is a frequent diagnosis blown up into a universal stereotype. Some suicides are suffering from what Freud first called misplaced aggression and later described as a diseased superego, but not all are. Universals of any kind are fantasies, not empirical realities. (The hypocrisy of the courts has also encouraged the dogma that suicides are unhinged.) It depends on the case.

Therapists deal only with the "attempteds," not the successful and thorough ones, and this gives a marked bias or skew to their speculations and theories. Even more speculative are the ideas of nonsuicides who have lively imaginations (Thomas Mann, Boris Pasternak), especially when combined with psychological jargon. Real suicides rarely leave any record, and even more rarely explain themselves in any reflective detail. There are only a few exceptions like Arthur Schopenhauer, who thought it through but did not do it, and Sylvia Plath, who did. We only have to read Lael Wertenbaker's *Death of a Man*, the story of her husband's noble and sane decision to cheat cancer of its terminal insults, to get a more realistic appreciation of what suicide can be.

The basic issue is whether quality of life is more valuable than life *qua* life. Any defense of suicide has to opt for quality, not quantity. The sacralists, those who invest life with a sacred entelechy of some kind, make all direct control by humans over their lives taboo. (We can see this in the abortion debate as well as in the question of suicide.)

Those who promptly and dogmatically put being alive as the first-order value need to reappraise their ethics. One's life is a value to be perceived in relation to other values. [At best it is only *primus inter pares*.] Without life, other things are of no value to us, but by the same token, without other things, life may be of no value to us. In *The Tyranny of Survival* Daniel Callahan puts it succinctly. "Unlike other animals, human beings are consciously able to kill themselves by suicide; some people choose to die." They want more than "mere survival," he thinks. "Models which work with ants do not work well when extrapolated to human beings."

And the reason for this, we can add, is that human beings, unlike purely instinctual creatures, do not regard life as an end in itself. Life to be up to human standards has to integrate a number of other values, to make it *worth* our while. Truly human beings can choose to die not only for reasons of love and loyalty, but just because life happens to be too sour or bare. In Sean O'Casey's words, a time may come when laughter is no longer a weapon against evil.

The *ethical* problem, how to make value choices, comes down, as we have seen, to whether we reason with or without absolutes of right and wrong. Bayet back in 1922, in his *Le Suicide et la Morale*, said there are two kinds of approaches: an ethic of *a priori* rules and taboos and universal prohibitions, or, alternatively, a *"morale nuancée,"* an ethic rooted in variables and discrimination, trying to judge acts by their consequences, *a posteriori*. The appraisal made here is built on moral nuances.

Socrates and Karl Jaspers, twenty three hundred years apart, thought that the business of philosophy is to prepare us for death. Religionists, in their own way, have taken hold of that task; they have tried to cope with it by a denial maneuver in the form of promising eternal life. Philosophers have ignored it for the most part. Still, a good start was made with Epictetus' dictum, "When I am, death is not. When death is, I am not.

Therefore we can never have anything to do with death. Why fear it?'' In present-day terms we have Camus's opening remark in his essay, *The Myth of Sisyphus*, that there is ''but one truly serious philosophical problem, and that is suicide.''

We have a striking paradigm for the ethics of suicide. In his *Notebooks 1914-16* Wittgenstein said that suicide is the ''elementary sin''—blandly assuming, in tyro fashion, that survival is the highest good, even though it is individually impossible and corporately improbable. On that basis he declared that ''if anything is not allowed, then suicide is not allowed.'' But very quickly his superb mind forced him to add: ''Or is even suicide in itself neither good nor evil?'' Exactly. Right there, in a phrase, is the whole point ethically. Nothing is in itself either good or evil; neither life nor death. Quality is always extrinsic and contingent.

The full circle is being drawn. In classical times suicide was a tragic option, for human dignity's sake. Then for centuries it was a sin. Then it became a crime. Then a sickness. Soon it will become a choice again. Suicide is the signature of freedom.

Fifteen

Experiments on Humans

In March, 1976, I read a paper at a World Health Organization conference in Geneva on the individual and the community in relation to research and testing of drugs. I began with an ethical premise, namely, that as moral agents we all have a right and an obligation to restrict or prohibit anybody's freedom to harm others, unless it be for the sake of the general welfare or a proportionate good.

SCOPE OF INQUIRY

The qualifying clause in this premise fits discussions of most human problems, such as foreign or civil war, the punitive and preventive coercions of law enforcement, social security legislation, and the delivery of health care. In the present context, however, scientific research and clinical trials in medicine specifically will be in mind. The development and use of complex biological substances and agents (globulins, serums, vaccines, antitoxins, antigens) are an important sector on the experimental front. Remarkable work is being done, even at such basic levels as the use of interferon to combat viruses.

Primary ethical concepts, however, apply broadly enough to cover synthetics as well as biologicals. There is no peculiar or idiomorphic system of ethics for research in biologicals alone. Furthermore, we ought to include the investigators themselves and prospective beneficiaries of the research as among the human beings who are involved, and who have moral claims to be considered along with the claims of research subjects (therapeutic and nontherapeutic). These parties to the process are too often treated as faceless or actually nonexistent.

The moral principles of research and investigative medicine have loomed larger since modern medicine got its start, with a shift from the spirit of Galen, relying on tried and true remedies, to the spirit of Paracelsus, i.e., the philosophy (a cognition theory) that experience is more important than tradition. It was this shift that loosed pharmacology's genius for scientific inquiry and experiment.

We have already noted the difference between the medical model of Aesculapius (a one-to-one obligation between physician and patient) and the one upheld by his daughter Hygeia, based on prevention as well as therapy, in the public interest as well as in the interest of private health.

The imperatives of social ethics have first claim on us; that is my basic contention. The Hippocratic Oath spoke only of a physician's obligation to his patient. The Helsinki Declaration (1964) still held to the doctrine that "my patient's" needs get first consideration, although it then adds a vague duty "to safeguard the health of the people." Therein lies the problem. Usually the tension between personal and social interests can be compromised, but when there is an irresolvable conflict or true dilemma (if one or the other must be chosen), we ought to prefer the good of the greater number.

Such at least is the baseline of this paper, even though it stands somewhat against the traditional Judeo-Christian preference for the inviolability of the individual. It is the same basic premise as in the military draft, sacrificial acts of heroism and martyrdom, confiscation by eminent domain, or traffic signals at intersections. The public *versus* private interest seeps into everything.

"What can we do about this agonizing dilemma?" Walsh McDermott once asked. "Obviously we cannot convene a constitutional convention of the Judeo-Christian culture and add a few amendments to it. Yet, in a figurative sense, until we can do something very much like that, I believe deeply that the problem, at its roots, is unsolvable and that [in biomedical ethics] we must continue to live with it." For the present, Dr. McDermott thinks, we are just coping with it by reciting our ambiguous Oaths and Declarations in the accents of hypocrisy, "that marvelous human invention by which we are enabled to adapt to problems judged to be not yet ripe for solution."[1]

Martin Arrowsmith, the bacteriologist in Sinclair Lewis's novel, went off as a disciple of Hygeia to an island in the Caribbean during an epidemic of plague, taking a new bacteriophage to test its safety and efficacy for preventive medicine. It was a unique opportunity, yet, in the situation, Arrowsmith ruined it because he felt he could not withhold the product from a randomized control group.[2] Was his compassion ethical? He himself was unable to say. His friends and fellow scientists, Gottlieb and Sondelius, were sure it was unethical. Here is a searching question: Is it susceptible of an answer?

How are we, then, to relate such hypothetical situations to historically real situations such as the Tuskegee syphilis study? This long-term investigation of untreated syphilis in a group of black men in six Southern states started in 1932. It was conducted under the auspices of the United States Public Health Service to determine the course of the infection. Even after both penicillin and heavy metals became available in the forties this longitudinal study was not interrupted, nor were the subjects informed of the new armamentarium. The affair was not uncovered until 1972. It was then promptly condemned by a panel set up by the Department of Health, Education, and Welfare, which included people from medicine, law, religion, labor, and government.[3]

As William Curran said, "It is difficult to quarrel with any of the substantive conclusions of the ad hoc panel."[4] Inquiry showed that the program had not provided for informed consent, that it lacked a written protocol, had no assurances of reliability, had no data base, and also was very questionably designed. This is an overwhelming indictment, both ethically and scientifically. But, we should ask, what if the scientific protocol had been acceptable, yet the efficacy of the antibiotic subsequently developed had remained still undemonstrated? In this situation would silence as to the penicillin have been ethical (i.e., justifiable) in the interests of a double-blind experiment? (Asking "what if" questions is an important tool of ethical analysis and criticism, as it is of decision-making theory.)

Without getting bogged down in detail or being unnecessarily analytical, let me just list, by title only, some fifteen distinguishable factors generally recognized, which enter into the total mix of the ethics of the research, development, and use of biologicals. The fifteen factors are: risk (for both subjects and investigators), avoidance of harm (*non nocere*), reportage (professional probity), prehuman tests (animal studies), consent (competence as to freedom and information), benefit (proportionate good to be gained), avoidance of deception (of subjects), design (scientific standards), privacy (confidentiality), motivation of participants (both subjects or investigators), cost (part of risk-benefit calculations), fraud (deception in reporting), in-course cancellation (by subjects or investigators), monitoring, and review (peer and public). There is a voluminous literature extant dealing with the ethics of research; it shows a fairly impressive consensus on some scores and very little agreement on others.

Five of these features or factors have become threadbare ethical issues, nearly talked or argued to death. They are: consent, privacy or confidentiality, avoidance of harm, fraudulent representation, and duress. By this date they are problems of enforcement, no longer serious ethical questions. Seven other aspects need sharper scrutiny and more rigorous appraisal: *risk-benefit calculations*; when *investigators* should be *subjects*; cancellation or *withdrawal*; *public* as well as peer *review*; *costs in relation to resources and need*; *liability* for injuries to subjects; and guidelines for the *selection* of both subjects and investigators.

All of these matters are more easily settled on the small scale of clinical experimentation than on the large scale of test populations. Complexity grows as we move from *in vitro* to animal to human tests, and also as we escalate from using 10-100 to 100-300 to 300-30,000 subjects at the human level.

In semi-scholastic circles reference is often made to a conceptual construct known as The Ideal Observer, originally put together by Roderick Firth.[5] This ideal moralist has five traits with which to weigh problems of right and wrong: he is omniscient—knows all the relevant facts; omnipercipient—can imagine all the human feelings involved; disinterested—is impartial and without self-interest; dispassionate—free of emotional bias; and consistent—uses generalizable principles to fit similar situations. But the most important thing about him is that he does not exist. Real human beings are only finite creatures, in all respects.

Two unusually candid papers on biomedical ethics are worth mention, one by Daniel Greenberg[6] and the other by Danner Clouser.[7] They both take a sharp look at some reasons for the backlash or negative reaction to the build-up ethics has had in the past ten years in science and medicine. Greenberg speaks of "that loose amalgamation of anxieties and passions that comes under the banner of medical ethics." Clouser is the professional ethicist of the two, however, and we can profit if we examine the way he treats the question. (I endorse his analysis. To demythologize ethics is not to downgrade it.)

Professor Clouser suggests at least eight things to be confessed about what the ethicist can or cannot contribute to moral decision-making. (1) Medical ethics offers nothing new, only ethics attempting to function in a new area of interst. (2) It employs notions "we ordinarily acknowledge in everyday life," and this is the case also with its "reasoning about the medical-ethical issues . . . " (3) We cannot expect the ethicist (ethician?) to be accepted as "the expert" since "what the professional ethicist does is not different in kind from what we all do in deliberating about a moral issue." (4) It is also noteworthy that "a serious limitation. . . is that ethics is a fairly blunt instrument; it does not cut finely." Therefore "it does not determine one or only one action that receives the moral seal of approval"; most commonly "all of the possible actions infringe on one moral rule or another, in which case it is a matter of choosing what one regards as the lesser evil."

Clouser's confession continues: (5) Ethics helps "structure" the moral issues of medical science and treatment but this does not "necessarily mean making a decision on what to do in the situation." (6) Often "the field really is not narrowed down much by moral criteria, and frequently the decision is ultimately made on the basis of some belief, predilection, or matter of taste." (7) Ethics has to have "outside" help. Pivotal decisons "such as 'normal,' 'rational,' 'sick,' 'person,' 'competent,' and 'voluntary' need considerable conceptual analysis by a variety of specialties," as well as empirical help with risks, the effect of drugs on judgment, physical and psychological reactions to information, and the like. Finally, he concludes that (8) "for the most part" we have to work our morals problems out "by trade-offs, compromises, convincing arguments, or whatever, so that the interests of all of us will be served as far as possible." (This "ethicist's confession" is strikingly pragmatic, utilitarian, relativistic, and pluralistic.)

So much for a professionally sophisticated assessment of the role of ethics in biomedical problems. There is, however, a more positive side, given Clouser's reservations. We may believe, as the editor of *The New England Journal of Medicine* does, that knowledgeable ethicists can sometimes help doctors and investigators to grasp more fully the value alternatives and spread of options between which they will have to choose, even though we rule out those ethicists who are "more activists than philosophers" and "too ready to act as self-appointed judges in labeling this or that medical research activity as 'unethical'." This he calls "the unethical in medical ethics."[8]

We seem to be saying in effect that ethics is no more than informed common sense. Very well, let us say so; that is what it is. Ethics deals with what we happen to hold to be good, and right actions are what conduce to the good—to what we "value." We approve human acts ("moral value") and things ("nonmoral value") for personal and cultural reasons, for subjective as well as objective reasons. At the most, we might *justify* them; we cannot verify them. Ethics is not a true-false discipline. There is no way to "prove" it is wrong to steal; we can only assert it is wrong (usually but not invariably being able to justify our judgment). The end product of the ethical process, as of legal or judicial thinking, is a judgment, not—as in science—a conclusion. Deciding whether something is good or evil is not a problem in verification or falsification. We can only approve or disapprove ethical opinions.

In saying that ethics is informed common sense, we ought not to ignore the fact that common sense is not always so commonly come by, and neither is adequate information. Even if ethics deals with value determinations and preferences subjectively, there are nonetheless things to be known about options, about frequencies and likelihoods, and about the history of human experience with them. The only alternative to this theory of ethics is to believe (a) that there is an objective moral order, and furthermore (b) that this moral order is known by special revelation (as in a religious faith system) or by reason somehow amenable to occult verification. Research scientists and medical investigators naturally prefer to be rational rather than metarational, to check their value perceptions against those of others, and to be as coherent and responsible as possible when making their decisions.

Medical research is inevitably and properly surrounded by regulations, established both from within and without professional circles. This is not, however, an unmixed blessing. In the world today there is a mood of suspicion and dislike for science and technology, in the affluent and developed countries rather than in the undeveloped countries. Its causes are probably a mixture of anger and fear because of various misuses of science and technology (especially of technology), combined with jealousy and envy of the learning, training and competence behind them. Many of the ethical principles upon which the regulations are based explicitly or implicitly are contained in the Nuremberg Code, the Helsinki Declaration of the World Medical Association, and (in the United States) the American Medical Association's Guidelines for research; and, we should add, the 1969 Regulations of the United States Public Health Service.

There are well-publicized instances of unethical practice. Not only the Tuskegee case but the New York cancer cell study, the thalidomide disaster beginning in 1960, the hepatitis infection of soldiers in World War II from pooled human plasma in a live virus vaccine, even the Elixir Sulfanilomide affair back in 1937 (using untested diethylene glycol as a solvent). The full list would be a long one.

As an ethicist I am sensitive to the fifteen different ethical factors I have listed above. At the same time, knowing that there are no "ideal observers" and no "moral experts" (*vide* Clouser), and that moral judgments are only blunt instruments bringing ethical issues down in the end to trade-offs and compromises of a common sense kind, I am wary of promoting too many ethical "principles" too finely drawn.

There is much practical wisdom and ethical perception in the position of the Public Health Service in the Southam-Mandel cancer study exposé. Agreeing positively that moral standards and ideals are imperative, they still thought that "proper ethical and moral standards are more effectively guarded by the process of review and criticism than by regulation."[9] In other words, situational or case-by-case decisions are better than rigid *a priori* rules. Professor Wolfensberger's classic survey of research ethics unfortunately used the language of "rules" and "codes," yet his intention was certainly not to drag us from conscientious guidelines (principles) into moralistic inflexibility and paralysis.[10]

Under pressures from powerful sectarian elements, the National Institutes of Health in 1974 slipped temporarily, for a year of so, into a taboo kind of ethics on fetal research. This telltale episode combined politicization of medical science, similar to Lysenko's distortion of genetics in the Soviet Union, and doctrinization similar to the Galileo tragedy in the history of Italian astronomy. For the sake of both ethical and scientific integrity, they would have been better advised to keep faith with the Livingston Report of 1964: "NIH is not...to assume an exclusive or authoritarian position concerning the definition of ethical boundaries or conditions mandatory for clinical research."[11]

We would all be immeasurably better off if investigators and their funding auspices, both public and private, would keep all rules based on moral values to a minimum, taking a laissez-faire stance toward research enterprises except when they hold both real and present dangers. Dangers to be avoided should be significant rather than minor or petty, and actual, not just possible (as in a slippery-slope argument about what conceivably *might* happen in the future). "Dangers" are dangers, of course, for all human beings—subjects, investigators, bystanders, present or prospective patient populations, and the general public.

One editor of a medical journal wrote in warning terms of a growing "ethical bureaucracy," to be discerned in the *Federal Register* reports: local institutional review committees, consent committees for certain research programs (e.g., involving prisoners, children, *ex utero* fetuses, the mentally ill), an NIH Ethical Advisory Board to advise funding agencies, a new National Commission for Protection of Human Subjects of Biomedical and Behavioral Research to promulgate ethical regulations, and finally, of course, Congress itself. "The number of inspectors threatens to outnumber the inspectees," with the possibility that "eternal ethical verities" will be determined by six-to-five votes.[12] (One ethical issue was actually settled by the National Commission with a five to four vote—two members absent.)

Setting aside "eternal ethical verities" as a presumably jocular reference, we can agree that each of these watch-dog bodies is appropriate in a
democratic society, yet also sounding a warning that "eternal vigilance"
is needed to protect science and medicine from the subverting interfer-
ences of pressure groups, doctrinal sectarians, bandwagon agitators, and
those whom Franz Ingelfinger calls simplistic "finger pointers," too
often inspired only by yesterday's gross misdeeds or ignorant of the
benefits to be gained from an experiment today. Public policy tends, as
Reinhold Niebuhr remarked, to be "a twilight zone where ethical and
technical issues meet." Science and medicine are only beginning to learn
how to deal with "public ethics"—the hard way, empirically.

The heart of ethics is obligation. To whom is it owed and how is it to
be rendered or fulfilled? Perhaps we need only to remark that valid
moral claims exist not only for subjects, but for investigators and society
too, and, therefore, what we owe morally to any one of these three
parties to medical research can be determined only in relation to the other
two. So-called rights are paired with commensurate "duties." It is true
that scientists and society owe subjects care and concern, but subjects
owe it to investigators and to society to help. We must reject the moral
opinion of Hans Jonas that "no one, not even society, has a shred of a
right" to ask anybody to take a risk for research—that volunteering is
absolutely "*gratia gratis data.*"[13] Investigators and subjects, both, owe it
to society to learn how to save life; but society owes them, each in his
own role, financial and legal support, and protection of their results
from abuse by business or yellow journalism. Investigators in particular
are morally obliged to serve societal priorities, to minimize risk and
harm, to welcome evaluation and review, to report fully, to accept
monitoring by their peers—but not by incompetent public watch-dogs
who are not equipped to watch intelligently.

As a parenthesis, I suggest that in a full-dress appraisal of medical
research we ought to take a hard look at one much neglected side of risk.
It would be easy to wax cynical about the virtual absence in the literature
of any discussion recently concerning the obligation of investigators to
volunteer themselves as experimental subjects. The silence is remarkable
when we recall Walter Reed in his yellow fever studies, the way J. B. S.
Haldane and his father before him frequently acted as their own subjects,
how Carrion innoculated himself with Bartonella bacilli to find a cure for
verruga peruana. Pettenkoffer and Emerick swallowed cholera bacilli,
Bergioni and Warneri and Lindemann submitted to injections of syphilis
organisms.[14] Sir John Eccles and his students self-tested in New Zealand
between 1944 and 1951.[15] If we speak of moral obligation, what of this

one? We can be sure that a rigorous analysis here would go a long way towards ethics in depth on the problem of research with human subjects.

There are three fundamental questions in ethics which need to be squarely faced by every one of us before we can make much headway with the questions at stake in research ethics. They have to do with (a) what we hold to be the highest good, (b) what method of conscientious decision making we should use, and (c) how we are to balance the individual interest versus the common interest. Let me take them up briefly, in a down-to-earth fashion and in the order given.

In current rhetoric we speak of value and values rather than of "the good" and particular goods. In either lexicon we mean what is regarded as desirable, among moral and nonmoral entities. Without being arbitrary or too reductive, can we not say that science and medicine are committed to humanism—the ethical first-order value of human survival and well-being, both individually and collectively? This is their *summum bonum* and their highest or ultimate criterion of what is worthwhile.

For some people humanism is theistic (having a divine sanction), for others it is naturalistic (no supernatural reference), but all are committed to the humanist standards. From this follows our obligation to protect subjects, to volunteer for tests and trials, to make choices maximizing or optimizing human health, to investigate and know how to do so.

It is occasionally said, somewhat abrasively, that science as such has "truth" as its highest good and its only obligation. (Science deals with truths, not with *the* truth.) Yet the search for knowledge is for the sake of human beings, not the other way around. Human interest has the first-order priority.

It was for this reason that scientists in 1974 called a moratorium on research with recombinant DNA molecules or plasmids, as a biohazard. They thought a drug-resistant carcinogenic construct might get loose and threaten both scientists and society at large. Only when the Asilomar conference, "on the risks and benefits of recombinant DNA research," agreed on various containment procedures did the research get a renewed "proceed with caution" signal. For this same reason, work on bacterial warfare at Fort Detrick, Maryland, was shut down permanently. "Forbidden experiments," because of "dangerous knowledge," are conceivable, if the dangers are found to be both real and present enough to justify suspending the scientific "habit of truth." The question always is, how real and how present is "enough," and resorting to bans to evade the burden of decision is a moral evasion.

The work of ethics in biomedical research, then, is critically to evaluate all investigations by the measure of the humanist principle, a humane or humanitarian yardstick, checking them out for the values of health, happiness, professional vocation, scientific discipline, and social well-being. These are the parameters within which to evaluate a protocol on the fifteen ethical factors we have listed.

In this world of relativities, decision means having to choose between values. Looking at the risk problem, Walter Modell once pointed out that "as there is no drug without hazard, there can be no testing of new drugs without risk."[16] This is why the law allows the dangerous Pasteur treatment for rabies; in the common law it is an "unavoidable" life-saving risk using an unsafe biological product. The Department of Health, Education, and Welfare allows "minor" but no "substantial" risks to subjects in research. These terms are (probably wisely) not spelled out, of course, and if there were a scale of risk, it would have to be stepped alongside a scale of benefit to be ethically significant. Decisions involve choices—less of this for more of that. The only realistic strategy of medical research is to reach a more favorable ratio between the probable adverse effect of experiment and treatment, and the probable adverse effect of disease.

"A man must judge whether an action is ethical or unethical in advance," said Marshall Walker, "hence he must try to predict the consequences."[17] Walker went on to describe what an ethical decision maker does: "He extrapolates his knowledge of the past to predict the future. This procedure is the domain of science. His classification of acts as ethical or unethical is as reliable as his scientific predictions of future events, no more and no less. Some ethical judgments will be as certain as, 'The sun will rise tomorrow'; others will be as uncertain as, 'the probability of rain tomorrow is three out of ten.' "

There are two ways to conceive of right conduct. In one view it means obeying and following moral laws already promulgated (by gods or churches or governments or hospitals or guilds or some other rule-making authority). The other view is to examine alternative courses of action to choose the one with the most good consequences. The ethics of most scientific workers, fortunately for mankind, are consequential. Few of them conduct their affairs by code morality or codified conduct. The survey of ethics and research with human beings by Professor Jay Katz of the Yale Law School and his colleagues is consequential throughout, although with no expressed awareness of it.

Professional ethical "codes," so called but misnamed, are actually quite flexible in the sense that they consist of guidelines and standards without fixed rules that allow of no exceptions. For example, informed consent is set out as a standard in United States government guidelines for the investigative use of new drugs, but there is no way to absolutize it if consequences and situational variables are taken into account. Therefore, the official full statement is "except where they deem it is not feasible or, in their professional judgment, contrary to the best interests of such human beings." If no discretion was possible and "the right thing to do" was prefabricated (thus ruling out moral decision-making, in effect), there would be no responsibility—only obedience. Unable to be Kantian, with categorically imperative rules, science and medicine act consequentially, for the sake of humane results.

Instead of "commandments," then, medical science needs guideline principles, and only as many as ethical practice requires. "The scientist escapes lightly—instead of ten commendments only four," said Bentley Glass. He gives them: "To cherish complete truthfulness; to avoid self-aggrandizement at the expense of one's fellow-scientist; fearlessly to defend the freedom of scientific inquiry and opinion; and fully to communicate one's findings through primary publication, synthesis, and instruction."[18] I would add a fifth: to have concern for all persons involved, not only subjects, but investigators and prospective beneficiaries.

To repeat an observation made in another place, I agree with a past editor of *The Journal of the American Medical Association* who advised us succinctly to decide moral questions according to the case or situation, rather than by universalizing rules and laying down categorical prohibitions. The wisest ethical method is situational; nondogmatic, flexible, particularized, value-oriented. Dr. Ingelfinger complained, after a National Academy of Sciences meeting on "Experiments and Research with Humans: A Conflict in Values," that some of the ethicists "insisted that the care of patients should be the result of categorical absolutes, that a balance of risks and benefits should play no role. How abysmally ignorant of medical practice is such a position! It was all very disheartening."[19]

The so-called Nuremberg Code set out after the trials of the Nazi prison camp experimenters has supplied the core of current ethical considerations. It had ten basic principles only: on consent, results otherwise unattainable, proportionate risk and benefit, animal pretesting, avoidance of harm, avoidance of fatal effect, professional qualifications, the rights of subjects and investigators to withdraw, termination if subject is in jeopardy, and stopping if fatal consequences are foreseen (except when the experimenters are also the subjects).

At the hearings of *United States versus Karl Brandt*[20] an American physician was asked: If a city is dying of a plague and you have a drug you believe could save the populace, yet it has never been tested in a human subject, and the mayor says, "Here is a prisoner condemned to die and here is a man dying of cancer; try it out on them," would you do it? The doctor replied no, he would not. If he had agreed, would he be right? If the prisoner and the cancer patient refused to be subjects could we justify "using" them anyway? Can a cost-benefit or proportionate good case be made for it? How weighty ethically is "the greatest good of the greatest number"?

Obviously this utilitarian theory lies behind most of our legislation; it is the moral principle of legislation and laws in democratic societies. When we stop to think carefully, we know that we cannot approve of sacrificing the many for just one, or even for only a few. Experimental science is risking some lives to save more lives, and, in doing so, it has better reason than public safety policy, which sometimes sacrifices lives rather than spend the money for preventive measures.[21]

To be "impersonal" in the sense of counting heads is not in any sense to be antipersonal or nonpersonal. It is being multipersonal. It is preferring several or many persons over one or a few. Randomization of research subjects is still a very personal, very "human" procedure. To sacrifice the one for the many is to save many ones. The "greatest number" is not an abstraction; it is the sum and count of real, particular, and personal individuals. Counter to Edmond Cahn's judgment, if the Pharaoh was wrong to spend the lives of many workingmen (slaves?) to build the pyramids, it was not the loss of life that made it wrong; it was the poor balance of human life against piled stone.[22]

The ethics of medical care and medical research should see its problems broadly, socially, through a telescope—not just through a microscope. We will have to stop the myopic and often irresponsible escape from the agony of ethics, which we try to do in shibboleths like "my patient comes first" and "first come first served," and "medicine is not a social service." These unethical gambits are based on the Aesculapian model, not on the model of Hygeia, which is so much more appropriate to our highly interdependent modern world.

It is perfectly plain that ethical judgments are not simple; not black-or-white, either-or choices. It is also plain that decision makers, like it or not, are moral agents; value (ethical) considerations enter into decisions in everything, including research and investigative medicine. Ethics is a process by which a chooser, according to perceived values, comes to a decision about what he ought to do in a certain choice situation. The more we know, the better we can choose.

Furthermore, if we are not radical egoists and individualists, we will try to choose the good of the greatest number, the social interest. Our moral decisions then become matters of distributive or allocative justice, as in triage judgments. We have to calculate, count, measure.

Ethicists are not like the old-time doctors with a bag full of specific remedies; they do not have a "system" or armamentarium of specific moral rules, imperatives, commandments, prohibitions, and the like for specific questions of conscience. Their role, when moral problems arise in medicine and medical research, is more like that of the consultant or the monitor or the "friend of the court." They can be asked in to see if they can find or think of anything else that ought to be taken into account besides what is already perceived by those engaged in the work under scrutiny. They are resource people for decision makers, question askers rather than answer givers.

But good question asking is the key to answer getting and decision making in medical research and probably in anything else.

1. Walsh McDermott, "Opening Comments on the Changing Mores of Biomedical Research," *Annals of Internal Medicine* 67 Supplement 7, (1967), 39-42.

2. Sinclair Lewis, *Arrowsmith* (New York: Harcourt, Brace and Company, 1924).

3. Final report of the Tuskegee syphilis study ad hoc advisory panel (Washington, D.C.: United States Department of Health, Education, and Welfare, 1973).

4. William Curran, Law-medicine notes, *The New England Journal of Medicine* 269 (1973) 730-731.

5. Roderick Firth, "Ethical Absolutism and the Ideal Observer," *Philosophy and Phenomenological Research* 12 (1952), 336-341.

6. Daniel Greenberg, "Ethics and Nonsense," *The New England Journal of Medicine* 290 (1975) 321-322.

7. Danner Clouser, "Medical Ethics: Some Uses, Abuses, and Limitations," *The New England Journal of Medicine* 293 (1975) 384-387.

8. Franz Ingelfinger, "Ethics and High Blood Pressure," *The New England Journal of Medicine* 292 (1975) 43-44.

9. E. Langer, "Human Experimentation—New York Verdict Affirms Patient's Rights," *Science* 151 (1966) 666.

10. W. Wolfensberger: "Ethical Issues in Research with Human Subjects," *Science* 155 (1967) 47-51.

11. R. Livingston, Program report on survey of moral and ethical aspects of clinical investigation, Memorandum to Director, National Institutes of Health, November 4, 1964 (Washington, D.C.)

12. Franz Ingelfinger, "The Unethical in Medical Ethics," *Annals of Internal Medicine* 83 (1975) 264-269.

13. Hans Jonas, "Philosophical Reflections on Experimenting with Human Subjects," *Daedalus* 98 (Spring 1969) 222.

14. V. Veresayev, *The Memoirs of a Physician* (New York: Alfred A. Knopf, 1916), 365-366.

15. John Eccles, "Animal Experimentation Versus Human Experimentation, in Defining the Laboratory Animal," National Academy of Sciences (ISBN 0-309-01862-5), (Washington, D.C., 1971).

16. W. Modell, "Hazards of New Drugs," *Science* 139 (1963) 1180.

17. M.Walker. *The Nature of Scientific Thought* (Englewood Cliffs, New Jersey: Prentice-Hall, Inc., 1963), 153-156.

18. B. Glass: "The Ethical Basis of Science," *Science* 150 (1965), 1258.

19. Franz Ingelfinger, "The Unethical in Medical Studies," 269.

20. "The Medical Case," in *Trials of War Criminals before the Nuremberg Tribunals*, vols. 1 and 2 (Washington, D.C.: U.S. Government Printing Office, 1948).

21. G. Calabresi, "Reflections on Medical Experimentation on Humans," *Daedalus* 98 (1969), 387-405.

22. Edmond Cahn, "Drug Experiments and the Public Conscience," in *Drugs in Our Society*, ed. P. Tolalay (Baltimore: The Johns Hopkins Press, 1964), 255.

Sixteen

Recombining DNA

A reference earlier to the debate about recombinant DNA and objections to it provides a case for the study of the ethics of risk taking at the deepest level of life. DNA is the nucleus of the nucleus of the basic cells of organic life. The debate still continues, and promises to go on into the future: a serious issue of social conscience.

The controversy embraces not only research in recombinant DNA molecules, but also what use we might make of the knowledge it gains for us. The whole issue comes down in the end to an ethical question: *Ought* we (not *can* we) seek for and make use of ways to direct and control the genetic structure of biological organisms, including mammals, especially humans?

Those who reply in the negative take one or both of two different grounds for their objection. Some say that such controls are morally wrong on principle. They contend, in a slight paraphrase of a familiar advertisement, "It isn't nice to fool with Mother Nature." "Nature," says Robert Sinsheimer, "has developed strong barriers against genetic interchange between species," and he suggests that there are moral limits to our right to innovate biological controls, e.g. DNA recombinations, "beyond which we should tread most gingerly."[1] He is not too plain-spoken, but some take him to mean that we ought to stop.

Other prohibitionists rest their objection less on a theory of "natural order" and more on consequential grounds. They contend that the risks or hazards are so great that neither the search for nor the use of such basic genetic controls can be justified. George Wald puts it succinctly: "Potentially, it could breed new animal and plant diseases, new sources of cancer, novel epidemics...I fear for the future of science as we have known it, for humankind, and for life on the Earth."[2]

Those who reply in the affirmative build their case on an assessment of what we already know empirically and theoretically, on what we can project or extrapolate rationally, and on a cautious but palpable trust in the future of both science and man. Their position is part reason, part faith. Winston Churchill used to grumble that it is always wise to look ahead, but difficult to look farther than you can see. A risk-benefit judgment in favor of recombining DNA is made even though we have no very full information, as yet, about either the risks or the benefits. Splicing DNA might turn out to be a Pandora's box, they concede, but they refuse to entertain apocalyptic fears and visions. It is conceivable, they suppose, that there might be such a thing as Forbidden Experiments, but this, in any case, is not one.

The issue, be it noted, is not one of weighing measured or calculated margins of risk and benefit. It is much too early for that. We have some knowledge of the facts, some empirical data, but both schools of opinion—both those who favor the research and those who are opposed—have to tip the balance of their judgment with visceral (attitudinal) as well as cerebral (rational) argumentation. Even when we look at what we already know, there is no agreement as to its bearing on the issue. For example, prohibitionists contend that a given strain of *E. coli*, the common colon bacillus, could easily become pathogenic if it is hybridized, while proresearchers insist that it would not. It is obvious that more than objective knowledge is at work in this dispute. We might almost say that sentiments and values and dispositions of the will are not only at work but *dominant*. Neither side is anywhere near having what Sir Karl Popper calls a "falsifiable hypothesis."[3]

This debate got its start in the sixties when molecular biology and biochemistry reported results bearing on human reproduction. Human genetics had begun pointing beyond sexual to nonsexual or asexual capabilities, for example, *in vitro* fertilization and replication from somatic cells. A strong protest arose against "tinkering" with human genes, a protest which is now being raised against exploring bacterial genetic control. Recently we have seen a swing in the tactics of obstruction, full circle back again, from fear of just bacterial gene control to fear of human gene control. This reactive fear takes the form of anger at the very thought of "tinkering" with human beings or "human nature."

(Language is more important in ethical discourse than in scientific discourse because of the role semantics plays. In common usage certain words carry a negative connotation. The literature of biomedical ethics is filled with pejorative words like "engineering" rather than construction, "tinkering" rather than modifying, "manipulation" rather than control, "gadgetry" rather than technology, "potential horrors" rather than risks. These are crafty examples of wordcraft. They are logomachies, battles of words, rhetoric used to slant discussion.)

My own answer to our question is affirmative, *ceteris paribus* and given our present information. Yes, we ought to (a) do research on recombinant DNA molecules, and (b) use what we learn to exert genetic control over the health and quality of human beings. (In another place, I have discussed at length the ethics of designed genetic change in humans; I did so favorably.[4]) The focus here is primarily on the issue whether designed change in bacteria is ethical, and again it will be argued affirmatively.

The question about physical and biological "containment" or safety controls is a scientific problem. The question whether the research *ought* to be done is, however, an ethical problem. I am *assuming* that there ought to be containment, but let me add parenthetically that, even if it could be shown that containment is impossible, that alone or of itself would not undermine the case for doing the research.

There are two levels in any analysis of risk-benefit problems, the empirical and the logical-ethical. If you prefer, we could call them the factual and the value-choice levels. Since nobody's ethical reasoning is any better than his facts, I will look first at some of the relevant biological reasoning bearing on our question. Since scientists disagree among themselves, I am forced to enter where nonscientific angels should fear to tread. As a layman, like all other laymen, I have to listen as well as I can and reach conclusions as well as I can.

The potential risks of splicing DNA are said to be of two kinds. The first is infection, of plants and animals and humans, from novel organisms produced by recombination. The second—somewhat more speculative, with less hard data—is that recombination or biosynthesis across species lines, as from single chromosome prokaryotes to genetically complex eukaryotic organisms, will in the long run end in unforeseeable disaster, because it subverts evolution's natural course.

Bernard Davis in a brilliant paper breaks down the first or immediate risk into three probabilities: (1) the risk of producing a pathogenic organism, (2) the risk of its affecting laboratory workers, and (3) the risk of its spread out into the community, even epidemically.[5]

The evidence seems to give little support to the fear that novel organisms contrived experimentally can survive much beyond their experimental use. The K12 strain of *E. coli* from the human gut used in DNA recombination research is a case in point. There is every reason to suppose that all conceivable bacterial chimeras have already occurred "spontaneously" in nature and are still occurring—then dying. The hazard for laboratory workers is very low, when properly safeguarded, as we know from our daily dealings with many deadly pathogens. Looked at as a risk-benefit policy in the United States, up to 1961, there were 2,400 recorded cases of bacteriological laboratory infections with 107 fatalities, to be weighed in the scales against millions of lives saved as a consequence of the research.

As for the fear of starting an epidemic, the research in bacteriological warfare at Fort Detrick in Maryland, which Nixon ended by presidential order, shows that in twenty-five years of work with highly virulent pathogens there were 423 infections, without a single secondary spread outside the laboratory. Only 150 infections have occurred in the Center for Disease Control, of the United States Public Health Service, with only *one* transmission—to a spouse. In the five years since research began on recombinant DNA molecules, there has not been a single infection. As Dr. Davis says, "It is easy to draw up a scary hypothetical scenario, if one's imagination need not be limited by considerations of probability."[6]

The great majority of microbiologists think it is wise, on both empirical and ethical grounds, to forge ahead with recombinant DNA. They include those scientists who first explained the risks and who then helped NIH to work out guidelines for both physical and biological containment devices such as high-security P4 laboratories, and biological materials such as self-destruct experimental organisms.

What are we to say, however, to the second level of fear—the fear that this research will create long-term evolutionary dangers? Here we can see more than a hint of what Ruskin called the "pathetic fallacy"—attributing feeling and purpose and judicious wisdom to subhuman nature. When Erwin Chargaff speaks of "evolutionary wisdom" being violated by "the curiosity of a few scientists", he only invites the kind of sarcasm seen in Stanley Cohen's rejoinder that it is evolutionary wisdom which "gave us the gene combinations for bubonic plague, smallpox, yellow fever, typhoid, polio and cancer."[7]

Sinsheimer is the best, or at least the most respected, spokesman for the prohibitionists, although I have noticed that his objection is expressed by indirection rather than by positive opposition. He puts it this way: "Nature has developed strong barriers against genetic interchange between species...The search for knowledge has often been hazardous;

many explorers have faced great perils. Now the hazards can encompass the planet, and we must not continue to rely upon the resilience of nature to protect us from our follies."[8]

This use of the term "follies" begs the quetion, of course, which is whether it *is* folly. Sinsheimer here shows a highly mystical and apocalyptic posture; he reflects the cosmic anxieties of biblical prophets rather than the calculating perspective of risk-benefit ethics. He seems to have an almost pantheistic belief that when men do what nature does not do they are somehow demonic, inviting a kind of built-in nemesis. However, when people disagree about their perspectives on investigative questions of this kind, no matter how sophisticated they may be, their contention remains essentially and almost by definition a matter of *faith*, neither verifiable nor falsifiable.

The current DNA controversy in biology, as an episode in the history of ideas, is a form of the old and perennial "nature versus nurture" debate. Alternatively, we might call it the "natural versus artificial" debate, or even "chance versus control."

Man is a maker and a selector and a designer, and the more rationally contrived and deliberate anything is, the more human it is. Any attempt to set up an antinomy between natural and biological reproduction, on the one hand, and artificial or designed reproduction, on the other, is absurd. The real difference is between accidental or random reproduction and rationally willed or chosen reproduction. In either case it will be biologic—according to the nature of the biologic process. If it is "unnatural," it can be so only in the sense that all medicine is.

When dark visions of the future are the basis for asserting, "We no longer have the absolute right of free inquiry,"[9] it is in order, surely, to say that there are no absolute rights to begin with, but that speculation about the distant rise of inimical chimeras is far too speculative—and very questionable theologically, philosophically, and biologically. Utopias and dystopias both have a place in creative literature, but as such they settle nothing about the future, nor do they tip the balance either way in specific risk-benefit assessments.

Joshua Lederberg once had the *mot juste* for those who would stop the learning process, which is what is recommended by some participants in this controversy: "The suppression of knowledge appears to me unthinkable, not only on ideological but on merely logical grounds. How can the ignorant know what they should not know?"[10] It seems to me as a philosopher, not a scientist, that if we cannot foretell the consequences of gaining new knowledge, we cannot foretell the consequences of not gaining it either. This is what the know-nothing strategy discounts or ignores.

The expectable benefits of DNA research are considerable, but still finite. They include inserting new genetic information to correct genetic faults in the treatment of human diseases such as hemophilia, diabetes, Tay-Sachs, and the like; to design a new bacteria for quick dispersion of oil spills and other pollutants; to make drugs, to produce hormones and enzymes in greater quantity than nature allows, to improve and increase food crops by improving their nitrogen-fixing capabilities, to increase the supply of meat and dairy animals. These things are benefits; I do not know how long the list is.

Over against these benefits are risks. Are they finite too? Or are they infinite, so that our human species might not survive, nor even life on Earth? If the risks are incalculable, unmeasurable, is there any rational ground for supposing that infinite risks will prevail rather than finite risks? I think not. Clearly, the burden of proof lies on the apocalyptic visionaries. It makes more sense intuitively to see the risks as finite rather than infinite, perhaps chiefly because we have no experience with either cosmic disaster *or* a zero probability of disaster. I put my eggs in the rational basket, assuming risks and benefits to be finite, and their balance amenable to present or further investigation and experience. If we had a so-called Science Court in which such controversial issues were debated preparatory to advising the public, this is the way it would go.

Empirical reasoning does not, as such, take us to a conclusion, either pro or con. We also have to look at the question in the light of logic and the values with which we assess both costs and benefits.[11] Have we said anything thus far which might run afoul either of the rules of coherent reason or of what we hold to be desirable and undesirable? Logic is impersonal, values are personal. Are we sufficiently agreed about the values at stake to pursue this analysis? Have we a substantial range not only of values but priorities in common? Perhaps some of us assign very little if any value to the hoped for fruits of directed DNA molecule control, such as a new insulin (even a cure for diabetes), or eliminating hereditary enzyme deficiencies, or antigens to immunize against tumors. I regard such things as desirable. They become undesirable only when they fall to the losing side of a gain-loss balance.

Let me explain that I approach this analysis with three axioms. If you dissent from any or all of these premises, you might call my ethical judgment into question. (Unlike microbiology, ethics has no exquisite techniques for testing its theoretical hypotheses or models.)

The first axiom is that our highest good or first-order value is survival of the human race, as well as of existing populations. It would be a weird ethic, not to say an anti-ethic, which could accept nihilism as one of its options.[12] Our posterity has a moral claim on us for consideration, both as to its safety and as to its biological improvement. Survival of the species is presupposed in all ethical reflection; it is only man's existence that makes obligation meaningful; only man makes rational choices between competing values.

Second, I determine what is right or wrong, good or evil, according to whether the consequences of an act or policy, on balance, add to or detract from the aggregate human well-being. When immediate consequences are totally unforeseeable or unpredictable, rational ethical judgment is impossible. Ordinarily, of course, we have some perception of the consequences of what we decide to do.

When we try also to take remote consequences (subsequences) into account we are uncertain, at best, but not wholly in the dark, and therefore not irrational. As moral agents we cannot get off the ethical hook just because we never know the distant future. But in any case, to ignore consequences is irrational, which is irresponsible, which is unethical.

My third axiom is that risk of error and risk of harm are given and inescapable features of our finite human condition. There is no such thing as a zero probability. We have no reliable calculus of risk for new advances, but the more we learn, the more we can distribute our possibilities and choose between alternative courses of action. Absolute containment of microbes is like absolute zero or a perfect vacuum, an unattainable ideal. Nobody should say the risks of recombining DNA are nonexistent. We cannot prove a negative. On the other hand, we can negate the negation by scientifically acquiring data and experience with which to measure the risks and thus to assess whatever fears are expressed. (After all, we know how to live with risk-benefit. The United States accepts fifty thousand highway deaths per year for the sake of having automobiles. There is no reason at all to predict that DNA molecule research will entail anything like the damage the automobile carries. If we find out that it does, we can revise our assessment.)

It seems obvious that any debate about whether to do research, as distinguished from how to do it, is academic in the sense of not practical or realistic. Even though the Asilomar conference in 1975 on DNA risks was international in its makeup, there is no way to create a world consensus on this ethical issue. If there were, I am sure it would lean heavily in favor of going ahead. We can see this in such things as Britain's Williams report and the British program of twenty licensed research centers; in the United States guidelines issued by the National Institutes of Health; continuing Soviet work (less fully reported). The World Health Organization has given its admonitory support, and so has COGENE—the Committee on Genetic Experimentation of the International Council of Scientific Unions. No government anywhere has tried to prevent recombinant DNA experiments, even though some of them have set up safety regulations along a wide spectrum from very mild to very severe. The research will go on, we may be sure.

After all, work with DNA molecules is not complicated nor expensive, nor does it need highly elaborate laboratory equipment. Scientists on both sides of the issue point out that bright schoolboys will be doing it fairly soon. Chromosomal recombination is not arcane; it is no more repressible than any other scientific inquiry. If scientists anywhere in the world were to embrace the doctrine of ignorance and ban such research, they would paralyze themselves and their countries, just as Stalin and Lysenko did Soviet biology when they throttled genetics fifty years ago.

Like it or not, we are unable to undo history. We cannot retrace all the big and little steps by which we have already drawn the blueprint of living genes, the basic building plans of life. No control, no laboratory, no government can black out genetics from the map of human knowledge— in particular they cannot stop the splicing and reassembly of different karyoplasms.

This is not to say that a thing is right just because it is going to be done anyway. It is a fallacy to think that because we can do something, such as splicing DNA, we "therefore" ought to. It does not follow that because we can, we should. I am only saying it is being done and will be done. "Murphy's law" (if anything can go wrong, it will) is yet another example of fallacious thinking; doomsters find it very seductive. It converts a probability factor, by means of a *non sequitur*, into a certainty.

Here we have, once again, the slippery slope argument, the contention that because a thing is dangerous or carries negative potential it will be the entering wedge leading to the evil consequences, and therefore it ought not to be done. As a debating ploy it is sometimes called the camel's-nose-under-the-tent argument.

The relative weight of the good to be gained and the loss to be suffered is irrelevant in the wedger's mind; it has no weight even when the foreseeable good plainly outweighs the foreseeable evil. Those who use it conjure up a parade of horrors to reinforce their negative feelings. Some call it scare tactics—a psychological weapon, not a reasoned objection. It loses sight of the difference between the virtue of prudence and the paralysis of anxiety neurosis.

Prudence calls upon us sometimes to forego foreseeable benefits when weightier risks or losses are *probable*, but the slippery slope objectors demand that we forego courses of action in which negative potentials are only *possible*. The answer to it, a sufficient one, has always been given in the classical tradition of philosophical and theological ethics: *abusus non tollit usum*—the abuse of a thing does not bar its use.

DeWitt Stettin once discussed the merit of proposals to ban research, and suggested that when the issue is problematic there are two eminently sensible indicators, without which a ban would not be justifiable.[13] They are borrowed from high judicial reasoning. One is that there shall be a clear and unmistakeable danger; the other is that the danger shall be present, that is, that it should be here and now rather than a forecast of a speculative future. Neither of these criteria is satisfied by the opponents of recombinant DNA research or designed genetic change.

I remarked earlier that I am speaking my piece as one of the men on the street, John Q. Public, because, in the first place, the scientific community disagrees within itself, and, in the second place, because the risks and benefits of both bacterial and (prospectively) mammalian bio-synthesis go right to the vital interests of all mankind. Nuclear biology is just as Promethean as nuclear physics. This is why Rene Dubos asserts that mankind now has the "privilege and the responsibility of shaping his self" as well as his society and his future.[14]

Senator Javits puts it this way: "A scientist is no more trained to decide finally the moral and political implications of his work than the public . . . is trained to decide finally on scientific methodologies."[15] Decisions about setting priorities in biomedical research and weighing non-quantifiable costs and benefits are in fact political. Properly and inevitably they invite the whole body politic to the conference table, including—but not exclusively—the scientists.

The general formula I propose for our problem is a sensible maxim: *Dangerous knowledge is never half as dangerous as dangerous ignorance.* Lewis Thomas, in "The Notes of a Biology Watcher," expresses it better than I can:[16]

"Is there some thing fundamentally unnatural, or intrinsically wrong, or hazardous for the species, in the ambition that drives us all to reach a comprehensive understanding of nature, including ourselves? I cannot believe it. It would seem to me a more unnatural thing, and more of an offense against nature, for us to come on the scene endowed as we are with curiosity, and naturally talented as we are for the asking of clear questions, and then for us to do nothing about it, or worse, to try to suppress the questions. This is the greater danger for our species, to try to pretend that we are another kind of animal . . . and that the human mind can rise above its ignorance by simply asserting there are things it has no need to know. This, to my way of thinking, is the real hubris, and it carries danger for us all."

1. Robert L. Sinsheimer, "Recombinant DNA—On our Own," *Bioscience* 26 (October, 1976), 599.

2. George Wald, "The Case Against Genetic Engineering," *The Sciences* 16 (September-October 1976), 6-11.

3. Karl R. Popper, *The Logic of Scientific Discovery* (New York: Basic Books, 1958), 40 ff.

4. Joseph Fletcher, *The Ethics of Genetic Control* (New York: Doubleday and Company, 1974).

5. Bernard D. Davis, "Darwin, Pasteur, and the Andromeda Strain," in *Genetic Engineering, Human Genetics and Cell Biology*, Supp. Rpt. II, Com. on Science and Technology, U.S. House of Representatives, Serial KKK (Washington, D.C.: United States Government Printing Office, 1976), 251-269.

6. Ibid., 254.

7. *Time*, April 18, 1977, p. 33.

8. Sinsheimer, "Recombinant DNA," 600.

9. Sinsheimer, quoted by Davis, "Darwin, Pasteur, and the Andromeda Strain," 258.

10. Joshua Lederberg, "Orthobiosis, the Perfection of Man," in *The Place of Values in a World of Facts*, ed. A. Tiselius and S. Nilsson (New York: John Wiley and Sons, 1971), 174.

11. See Carl Cohen, "When May Research Be Stopped?" *New England Journal of Medicine* 296 (May 26, 1977), 1203-1210, a persuasive case for recombinant DNA research based on a purely logical analysis. He concludes: "There is no valid practical syllogism, having true premises, whose conclusion is that research into recombinant DNA should be stopped."

12. Some philosophers have spoken of the "tyranny of survival." See, e.g., R.A. Watson, "Reason and Morality in a World of Limited Food," in *World Hunger and Moral Obligation* (Englewood Cliffs, New Jersey: Prentice-Hall, 1977), 116-123. Watson contends that food should be shared even if it means the extinction of the species.

13. DeWitt Stettin, "Freedom of Inquiry," *Genetics* 81 (November, 1975), 415-425.

14. René Dubos, *So Human an Animal* (New York: Charles Scribner's Sons, 1968), 106.

15. Statement at a Fairlie House conference, "Biomedical Research and the Public," April 1-3, 1976.

16. Lewis Thomas, "Notes of a Biology Watcher," *New England Journal of Medicine* 296 (February, 1977), 324-328.

INDEX

Abortion, 3-4, 7, 11, 44, 82, 86-87, 95, 101, 108, 119-120, 132-138
Aesculapius, 43, 177, 187
Agapism (loving concern), xii, 9, 32-33, 46, 56, 73, 91, 146-147, 157.
Aiken, H.D., 71, 132
Allocation (of resources), 2, 7, 41-53, 62, 74, 173, 187
Allocide, 141 ff.
American Association for the Advancement of Science, 9
American Hospital Association, 44
American Medical Association, 1, 43, 45, 153, 181
Anomie, 15, 173
Anscombe, G. E. M., 29
Aquinas, Thomas, 34, 38, 134-135
Aristotle, 23, 34, 37, 44, 67, 134, 170, 172
Artificial, the, 16, 65 ff., 87 ff., 126, 194
Astronauts, 8
Augustine, Saint, 24, 25, 37, 134, 171
Axioms (ethical), 195-196

Baier, Kurt, 31
Balguy, John, 33
Bangladesh, 62
Baram, Michael, 90
Beadle, George, 80
Behavior control, 7-8, 22, 24, 85, 121
Bentham, Jeremy, 29, 48, 84
Berg, Alan, 63
Berill, N. J., 81

Bible, the, 9, 37, 46, 49, 60, 70, 150, 156, 170, 194
Black, Max, 29
Blanshard, Brand, 36
Boulding, Kenneth, 47, 51
Brain death, 16, 75-76, 88, 159-165
Brave New World, 86, 103, 121
Brody, Howard, 2
Browne, Thomas, 171

Cahn, Edmond, 50, 187
Callahan, Daniel, 47, 74
Camus, Albert, 173-175
Casuistry, 34
Cerebral function, 14, 16, 20-21, 134, 151, 159-165
Chance, 50
Chase, Stuart, 23
Chargaff, Erwin, 193
Childress, James, 50
Chimeras, 85
Church of England, 78
Churchill, Winston, 191
Clarke, Samuel, 33
Cleanthes, 170
Cloning, 83 ff., 90, 118, 191
Clouser, Danner, 179-180
Club of Rome, 49
Codiga Penal (Uruguay), 154
Cohen, Stanley, 193
Colombia, 154
Comfort, Alex, 9

Compton, Christian, 160
Computers, 47-49, 52
Condorcet, Marquis de, 57
Consent, 7, 73, 74, 94, 102, 137, 141
Consequences, 21, 36, 54, 61, 63, 81, 82
  ff., 94, 100, 119, 136, 145, 155, 185.
Constitution, U.S., 87, 97, 118, 125, 137
Contraception, 44, 48, 57, 63, 108, 113,
  167-168
Control, 8, 15, 24, 79 ff., 85, 91, 107 ff.,
  128, 119, 152
Cooley, Denton, 75
Cooper, I. S., 143
Cost-benefit, 8, 47, 102, 187
Crick, Francis, 91
Cunningham, B.J., 69
Cushing, Harvey, 72
Curran, William, 178

Daedalus, 126
Dante Alighieri, 167
Darwin, Charles, 10
Da Vinci, Leonardo, 68
Davis, Bernard, xi, 192 ff.
Definition, 37
Deontology, 32, 82, 156
Dewey, John, 28-29, 37, 94
Diderot, Dennis, 84
DNA, 90, 122, 184, 190-198
Donne, John, 166
Dorfman, Robert, 51
Dostoievski, Feodor, 49
Dubos, René, 9, 10, 127, 198
Dubzhansky, Theodosius, 9, 81
Durkheim, Emile, 172

Eccles, John, 183
Einstein, Albert, 50
Elective death (see Euthanasia)
Emerson, R. W., 66
Empedocles, 5, 43
Epictetus, 174
Epicurus, 23
Episcopal Theological School, xi
Eschatology, 13, 35, 67, 116, 169, 171,
  174
Ethics, 115-116, 123, 149, 179-181, 183,
  184; act, situation, case, xii, 2-3, 27-39,
  55, 63, 104, 112, 119, 147, 167, 186;
  biomedical, xii, 1-2, 12, 123, 158, 177
  ff., 192; relative, 7, 32, 37, 49, 101,
  117-118, 119, 121, 146, 185; religious,
  9, 36, 55, 63, 71, 81, 82, 94, 96, 116,
  137, 150, 168-169, 171, 177; social, 42,
  46, 54 ff., 91, 114 ff.
Ethimetrics, 41-53

Eugenics, 124, 126
Euthanasia, 7, 11, 140 ff., 149-158, 166
Ewing, A. C., 33
Experimentation (human), 97, 99, 176-
  188; criteria, 178-179

Fallacies: all-or-nothing, 114; capacity,
  81; faulty generalization, 121; natural-
  istic, 27, 37, 56, 167; necessity, 81, 103;
  pathetic, 193; potentiality, 97, 144; un-
  distributed middle, 109
Famine, 54-64, 91
Fateh, Abdullah, 161
Feeling (emotion), 12, 15, 22,
Fertility control, 54-64
Fertilization (*in vitro*), 7, 15, 80, 82-83,
  86, 100, 191
Fetuses, 11, 74, 86, 93-104, 132, 135-137
"Fifth World," 58, 63
Firth, Roderick, 179
Fletcher, John, 144
Fletcher, Joseph, xi-xii, 147, 150
Forrester, Jay, 52
Fort Detrick, 184, 193
Frankena, William, 147
Frankfurter, Felix, 107
Freud, Sigmund, 173
Freund, Paul, 131

Galen, Claudius, 5, 177
Galileo Galilei, 82, 182
Generosity, 55-62
Genetics (human), 2, 78, 79-91, 152, 192
Glass, Bentley, 186
God, 9, 29, 50, 77, 116, 119, 144-147, 149,
  150, 151, 157, 168
Goodwin, William, 57
Good, the, 27-39, 180-181
Goodlin, Robert, 102
Grand Mufti of Jerusalem, 136
Greenberg, Daniel, 179
Greene, Graham, 164
Gustafson, James, 83, 89

Haldane, J.B.S., 81, 183
Hamilton, Michael, 81
Happiness (utility), 20-26, 32, 59, 146
Hardin, Garrett, xi, 53, 59, 63
Hare, R. M., 29-30
Hargis, Billy James, 55
Harrington, Alan, 167
Harvard Medical School, 16, 135
Health, Education and Welfare, Depart-
  ment of, 99, 178-185
Healy, Edwin, 71
Hegel, Friedrich, 51

Hellegers, André, 96
Helms, Jesse, 120
Hemingway, Ernest, 167
Heraclitus, 18
Herodotus, 23
Hippocratic Oath, 1, 5, 96, 157, 177
Homer, 23
Howe, J. W., 58
Hulme, T. E., 10
Human Subjects, National Committee for
    Protection of, xii, 182
Humanhood, 7-18, 25, 88-89, 132 ff.,
    151, 162
Humanism, xi, 23, 32, 122, 147, 157, 168,
    184
Hume, David, 29, 171
Hume, D. M., 160
Hunter, Thomas H., xii, 13, 160
Huxley, Aldous, 80, 121
Huxley, Julian, 84
Huxley, Thomas, 9
Hygeia, 93, 177, 187

Icarus, 126
Individualism, 51, 95, 114, 116, 183, 187
Infanticide, 140-147
Ingelfinger, Franz, 102, 183, 184
Inovulation, 7, 82
Insemination, artificial, 7, 82
Interspecific donation, 76-77
Intuition, 34
Italian Council of Ministers, 16, 135

Jacobi, Karl, 56
James, William, 21, 22, 36
Jaspers, Karl, 174
Javits, Jacob, 198
Jesus, 69, 166, 171
Joad, C. E. M., 172
Johns Hopkins Hospital, 142
Jonas, Hans, 46, 183
Jonson, Albert, 48
Jonson, Ben, 166
Judaism, 67, 69, 170
Judgments (moral), 2, 4, 9, 51, 80, 180-
    181
Justice, distributive, 41-53, 54-64, 117,
    155, 187

Kant, Immanuel, 4, 33, 81, 116, 143, 168,
    186
Kantrowitz, Adrian, 11
Karnofsky, David, 150
Kass, Leon, 82, 87
Katz, Jay, 97, 185
Kelly, Gerald, 70

Kierkegaard, Soren, 45, 51
Klett, Joseph, 159
Kluge, E-H. W., 144, 146
Knowles, John, 42, 62
Koestler, Arthur, 163
Koran, the, 169-170

Law, 106-112, 117, 123, 127, 128, 141,
    156, 153-154, 156-157, 158, 159 ff.,
    172, 186
Leach, Gerald, 89
Lederberg, Joshua, xi, 84, 86, 96, 194
Leo X, 68
Lewis, C. S., 80
Lewis, Sinclair, 177
Living Will, 153
Lobotomy, 8
Lorenz, Konrad, 37
Lower, R. R., 160
Lundberg, George, 30
Luther, Martin, 45
Lynch, J. J., 71
Lysenko, Trofim, 182, 192

McCormick, R. A., 81, 83, 146
McDermott, Walsh, 177
McFadden, Charles, 71
MacLean, Paul, 163
McLuhan, Marshall, 66
McNamara, Robert, 60
Malthus, T. R., 57
Mann, Thomas, 173
March of Dimes, 113
Massachusetts General Hospital, 45, 69,
    161
Meadows, D. H. and D. L., 49
Means and ends, 32, 35, 80, 81, 86, 102,
    111, 120, 143, 155
Medawar, Peter, 11
Medical College of Virginia, 159
Melville, Herman, 167
Michigan, University of, 25
Mill, J. S., 4, 24, 49, 110-111
Modell, Walter, 185
Mondale, Walter, 89
Montaigne, Michel, 171
Moore, G. E., 29 ff., 35
Moral agent, the, 3, 9, 12, 32-35, 82, 102,
    187
Morison, Robert, 7

National health insurance, 42, 45
National Institutes of Health, 98 ff., 102,
    163, 182, 196
Natural law, 10, 138, 147
Nature, 10, 116, 190, 191, 194

Nazis, 109, 120-121, 133, 150, 186
Neo-Malthusianism, 57-64
Neo-Platonism, 43
Newborns, 2, 7, 11, 20-22, 142, 144, 157
Niebuhr, Reinhold, 183
Noldin, H., 70
North, Dudley, 41
Nowell-Smith, P.H., 31
Nuremberg Code, 93

Oates, Captain, 173
O'Casey, Sean, 174
O'Connor, T. P., 41
Ortega y Gasset, José, 10
Oxford Famine Relief, 60

Pappworth, M. H., 95, 102
Paracelsus, Aureolus, 5, 177
Pasternak, Boris, 173
Pasteur, Louis, 185
Paul, Saint, 67
Peanuts, 4
Pell report, the, 100-101
Persons, 11, 89, 93 ff, 113, 125, 132 ff.,
    137, 138, 141, 144
Peter Bent Brigham Hospital, 72
Petrovsky, Boris, 72
Petrucci, Daniele, 82
Petty, William, 41
Pinocchio, 34
Pius XII, 68-70
Plath, Sylvia, 174
Plato, 23, 29, 136, 170, 172
Pluralism, 98
Popper, Karl, 29, 191
Population control, 55 ff.
Pragmatism, 30, 35, 43, 83, 95
Professional Standards Review Organiza-
    tions (PSRO), 45
"Pro-lifers," 103, 113, 137, 144
Proportionate good, the, 36, 80 ff., 84,
    94, 102, 146, 155, 176, 187
Protagoras, 9, 149
Prudence, 103, 120, 124, 197
Psychosurgery, 2
Pythagoras, 5, 170

Quality of life, 2, 9, 11, 88, 96, 101,
    109 ff., 121, 150, 163, 175
Quakers, 63
Quinlan, Karen Ann, 165

Ramsey, Paul, 13, 83, 144
Rathbone, F. S. and E. T., 9
Reed, George, 74
Reed, Walter, 183

Resurrectionism, 67
Richelieu, Cardinal, 169
Riesman, David, 172
Right-to-Die laws, 158
Rights: human, 1, 17, 55, 60, 89-90, 95,
    99, 108 ff., 117-118, 122, 128, 133, 141,
    145, 168, 172, 183, 194; patients', 2, 44,
    46, 137
Risk, 1, 73, 94, 145, 179, 191-195
Rockefeller Foundation, 42, 49, 62
Roe v. Wade, 4, 95, 137
Rostand, Jean, 135
Ruskin, John 193
Russell, Bertrand, 29
Russell, Jack, 160
Ryle, Gilbert, 38

Sahel, the, 61
Samuelson, Paul, 51
Sartre, Jean-Paul, 30-37
Schoeck, Helmut, 16
Schopenhauer, Arthur, 174
Scientific Unions, International Council
    of, 196
Semantics, 8, 88, 112, 191
Seneca, Lucius, 170
Sewall, D. H., 160
Sex selection, 85
Shakespeare, William, 51, 153, 168
Shaw, G. B., 84
Sherrington, C. S., 9
Shinn, Roger, 49, 91
Shulz, Charles, 4
Sidgwick, Henry, 147
Singer, Peter, 54
Sinsheimer, Robert, xi, 91, 164, 190, 193
Situation ethics, xii, 2-5
"Slippery slope," the, xii, 30, 102, 120,
    182, 197
Sloan-Kettering Institute, 150
Smythies, John, 163
Socrates, 11, 23, 132, 174
Sophocles, 51
Soul, the 24, 67, 75, 96, 134, 136, 169
Soviet Union, 182, 196
Sri Lanka (Ceylon), 48
Stalin, Joseph, 197
Stanford-Binet tests, 12
Sterilization, 7, 44, 61, 108, 120
Stettin, deWitt, 198
Stevenson, R. L., 144
Suicide, 31, 141 ff., 154-155, 166-175
Supreme Court, United States, 4, 95, 99,
    128, 137
Syllogisms, 18, 29, 36

Taboos, 25, 68, 101, 103, 145, 156, 169, 170, 174
Taylor, G. R., 49
Technology, 13, 17, 46, 66
Temple, William, 13, 147
Tertullian, 134
Texas Medical Center, 20
Theobald, Robert, 47
Theology, 4, 9, 35-37, 38, 67, 69-71, 120, 136, 144, 155, 168, 174, 198
Thomas, Lewis, 198
Thoreau, Henry, 80
Tillich, Paul, 13
Toulmin, Stephen, 31, 38, 52
Trade-offs, 8, 26, 47, 49, 102, 180
Tragedy, 51
Transexualization, 7
Transplants (tissue and organs), 2, 65-78, 158, 163
Triage, 7, 187
Truthtelling, 31 ff., 35, 167, 184
Tucker, Bruce, 159 ff.
Twain, Mark, 11

Unborn, the 27, 106-128
U.S.S.R. Criminal Code, 154
U.S. Aid for International Development, 54
U.S. Public Health Service, 178, 181-182, 193
Utilitarianism, 23-24, 30, 35, 48, 83, 116, 147, 187

Values, 2, 8, 27-39, 41, 50, 83, 90, 101, 119, 122, 145, 167, 180, 184, 187, 195
Vermeersch, A., 70
Virgin birth, 90, 118
Virginia Bar Association, 160
Virtue, 27-39

Wadlington, Walter, 160
Wagner, Robert, xi
Wald, George, 191
Walker, Marshall, 185
Weaver, Warren, 49
Weber, Max, 28
Wells, H. G., 84
Wertenbaker, Lael, 174
Whittier, J. G., 150
Wilder, Douglas, 161
Williams, Richard, 160
Wittgenstein, Ludwig, 29, 38, 45, 167, 175
Wolfensberger, W., 182
World Bank, 60, 63
World Health Organization, 42, 106, 176, 196
World Medical Association, 96, 153, 181
Wrongful life, 125

Zeno (of Citrium), 170
Zoroaster, 25